Our Complete List of Workshops

Associate Safety Professional (ASP)	**Certified Instructional Trainer (CIT)**	**Certified Hazardous Materials Manager (CHMM)**
Construction Health and Safety Technician (CHST)	**Certified Industrial Hygienist (CIH)**	**Certified Safety Professional (CSP)**
Occupational Hygiene and Safety Technologist (OHST)	**Safety Management Specialist (SMS)**	**Safety Trained Supervisor (STS)**

Safety Trained Supervisor Construction (STSC)

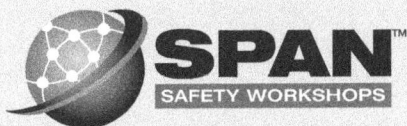

SPAN SAFETY WORKSHOPS

SPAN workshops offer proven techniques to help customers pass the exam the first time. The three day exam preparatory review course defines the scope of the exam; illustrates the complexity of problems to be encountered; reviews certification exam math, science and calculator skills; test strategy guidance; an overview of examine reference materials; and importance of a self-directed study program.

www.spansafetyworkshops.com

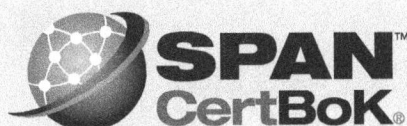

SPAN CertBoK®

An interactive, online Learning Management System (LMS). **CertBok**® delivers the essential knowledge required to successfully pass certification exams.

www.certbok.com

Dedicated to All Safety, Health and Environmental Professionals

Striving to Protect

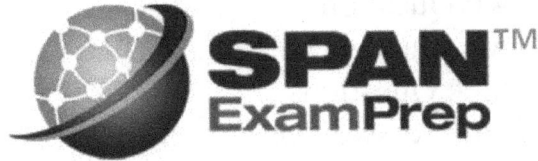

SPAN™ ExamPrep

www.spansafety.com

This Publication is not intended to guarantee that the user will pass an exam, become certified or in general may not cover every aspect of the certification process.

The information contained in this study workbook is intended to be used in preparation for the Construction Health and Safety Technologist® examination and should not be used as an authority in the professional practice of safety, health, or environmental compliance.

The Construction Health and Safety Technologist® (CHST®) Certification is a registered trademark of the Board of Certified Safety Professionals (BCSP). The opinions expressed are those of the authors and no guarantee, warranty, or other representation is made as to the absolute correctness or sufficiency of any information contained in this study workbook.

Daniel J. Snyder, Ed.D, CSP, OHST
Copyright © 2019 by SPAN™ International Training, LLC
402 W. Mt Vernon St #111
Nixa, Missouri 65714
Phone: 417 724 8348
info@spansafetyworkshops.com

ISBN 978-1-891017-70-4 (set)
ISBN 978-1-891017-68-1 (v.1)
ISBN 978-1-891017-69-8 (v.2)

Contents

Self-Assessment Exam One Questions

1) What is the purpose of metatarsal guards?
    A) Protect the insoles from puncture hazards.
    B) Protect the toes from crushing hazards.
    C) Protect the lower legs and feet from heat hazards.
    D) Protect the instep from crushing hazards.

2) Asbestos fibers and silica dust may cause a what effect in the lung tissue?
    A) Cystosis.
    B) Fibrosis.
    C) Necrosis.
    D) Scoliosis.

3) Respirators are generally divided into which of the following categories?
    A) Particulate and Supplied Air.
    B) Self-cleaning and Non-self-cleaning.
    C) Air-purifying and air-supplied.
    D) Gas Masks and Air Hoods.

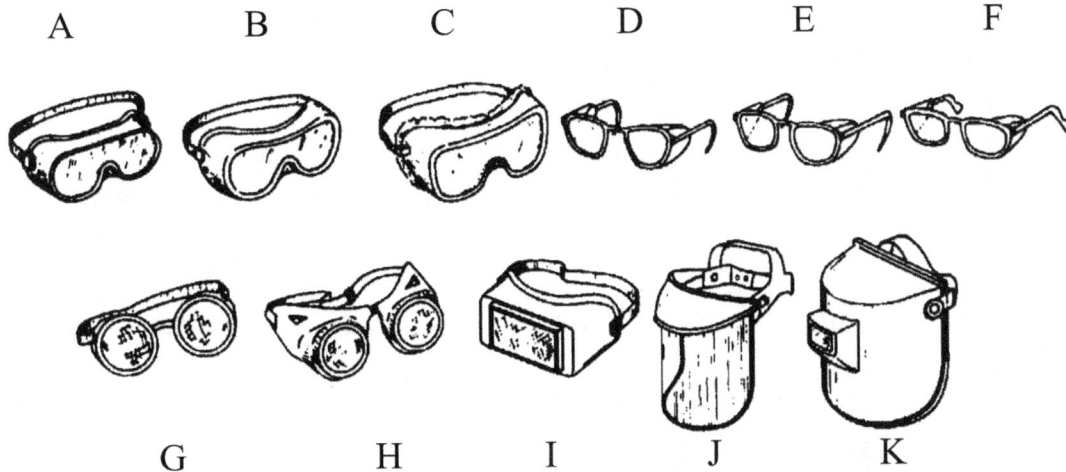

4) Using the illustration shown above which personal protective equipment would provide the greatest degree of protection and be the **most appropriate** for a worker doing heavy metal grinding?
    A) A & E.
    B) A, B or C and J.
    C) C & D.
    D) I or K.

5) A maintenance work station is located inside a hazard area for a robot, which is the **best** hazard control action?
   A) Place guarding around the workstation.
   B) Move the work station outside the hazard area.
   C) Conduct training for the maintenance department.
   D) Install a light curtain around the robot hazard area.

6) A full-face piece supplied air respirator in positive pressure mode has a protection factor of:
   A) 1000 APF.
   B) 100 APF.
   C) 10 APF.
   D) 10,000 APF.

7) According to an energy control program, it is required to ensure that before any worker performs servicing/maintenance on a machine or equipment, where the unexpected startup or release of stored energy could occur and cause injury, the machine or equipment shall be isolated from the energy source. This generally requires a physical lock and tag arrangement to meet the intent of the policy. When is it permissible to only use a tagout system of protection?
   A) If locks cost more than tags.
   B) On overlapping shift work.
   C) When other protective measures are in place.
   D) When the point of operation is higher than 7 feet above floor level.

8) In the welding environment the term *"GTAW"* represents which of the following?
   A) Gas Torch-Atomizing Welding.
   B) Gas Torch-Arc Waste.
   C) Gas Tungsten Arc-Welding.
   D) Gas Tungsten Atomizing-Welding.

9) What type of respirator should be used for entry into a confined space?
   A) Supplied air.
   B) Chemical cartridge.
   C) Charcoal filter.
   D) Airline with supplied escape bottle.

10) Which of the following respirator is an air-purifying type?
    A) Gas mask.
    B) SCBA.
    C) Airline respirator.
    D) Abrasive blasting helmet.

11) Which of the following is the **most correct** concerning a rigged load subject to the sudden movement of a hoisting apparatus (up or down) during a hoisting operation?
    A) The load should be padded.
    B) The load will not be affected.
    C) Stresses will be increased in the rigging.
    D) Safety factors are based on the increased stresses caused by such operations.

12) OSHA requires protective equipment for protection from high voltage electrical contact in some instances. These "rubber goods" consist of gloves, matting, blankets, hoods, line hose and sleeves. Several standards are available and cover initial/periodic testing and continued care and use of such equipment. Which of the following statements is **not** correct concerning electrical high-voltage gloves?
    A) Gloves must be given an "air" test prior to use.
    B) Rubber gloves are often worn with an approved leather outer glove.
    C) A metal reinforced outer glove should be worn over the rubber inner glove and the outer glove should be one inch longer than the inner glove.
    D) Periodic testing is necessary, the interval of such testing depends on the use of the glove and the conditions under which the glove is used.

13) When placing a standard straight ladder, the horizontal distance from the base to the vertical plane of the support should be approximately _____ the ladder length between supports.
    A) 1/3.
    B) 1/4.
    C) 1/2.
    D) 1/8.

14) Which of the following would be the **best** use of direct reading instrumentation?
   A) To determine the amount of several different hazards.
   B) To monitor for sporadic increases in a particular contaminate.
   C) To provide generalizations about several different gases.
   D) To provide absolute accuracy during the ongoing assessment of confined spaces.

15) A CHST is involved in a monitoring operation within an equipment repair area and is using a carbon monoxide direct reading instrument. The instrument has been reading 35 ppm for 4 hours, suddenly without any change in the conditions in the general area the indicator increases rapidly to 65 ppm and has remained constant for 5 minutes. Which of the following is the **most appropriate** action?
   A) Shut down the job site immediately.
   B) Quit monitoring.
   C) Continue monitoring.
   D) Stop and recalibrate instrument.

16) Which of the following selections is **not** true concerning portable wood ladder standards?
   A) Portable ladders cannot be coated or painted.
   B) Portable ladders must be constructed of high density wood and be free of sharp edges and splinters.
   C) Stepladders are limited to 20 feet in length.
   D) Single ladders cannot be longer than 30 feet.

17) All the following are instruments used to measure ionizing radiation **except?**
   A) Geiger Counter.
   B) Cutie pie.
   C) Condenser R-meters.
   D) Scatter Absorbers.

18) All the following requirements regarding types of scaffolds are correct, **except?**
   A) Guardrails and toeboards shall be installed on all open sides and ends of platforms more than 10 feet above the ground or floor, except needle beam scaffolds and floats.
   B) Scaffold erection is not permitted except under the direction of a competent person.
   C) Scaffolds must be built with a safety factor of 5.
   D) All planking used must be scaffold grade or equivalent.

19) Rolling tower scaffolds are popular with most of the trades, e.g.: painters, maintenance men, electricians, sign installers, heating and ventilating men, etc. The rolling tower is easy to move around in an area and provides a stable platform from which to work. Generally, these tower scaffolds are equipped with 5 or 8-inch casters that have a brake permitting the worker to lock the wheel. Additionally, the scaffold can be equipped with outriggers. Outriggers are required on any scaffold with a height to base ratio exceeding?
   A) 6.
   B) 5.
   C) 4.
   D) 3.

20) All of the following are requirements concerning the type and use of wooden planking **except?**
   A) Scaffold planking must be at least 1,500 psi fiber (stress grade).
   B) Scaffold planking shall be Scaffold Grade or equivalent.
   C) On a light duty scaffold (25 psf) the maximum permissible span for 2 × 10 nominal thickness lumbers are 8 feet.
   D) Bricks or cinder blocks are permissible for mud sills.

21) Substances that can damage the liver such as carbon tetrachloride, chloroform, tannic acid, and trichloroethylene are called?
   A) Nephrotoxins.
   B) Hematoxins.
   C) Hepatotoxins.
   D) Lacrimators.

22) In testing chemicals in the laboratory, toxicologists have learned that many chemicals act together in certain ways on biological systems. When the exposure to two different toxic chemicals produce a more severe effect than simply doubling the dose of either one alone, such as isopropyl alcohol and chloroform, is called?

    A) Additive Effect.
    B) Synergistic Effect.
    C) Potentiation.
    D) Antagonism.

23) The hepatitis B virus infects the liver. In some individuals, it develops into serious or fatal problems, such as cirrhosis, liver cancer, or chronic liver disease. Some people have no problems or symptoms yet become carriers of the virus. Which of the following represents the proper acronym for hepatitis B virus?

    A) HIV.
    B) HCV.
    C) HBV.
    D) HAV.

24) Which of the following **best** describes the function of barrier cream?

    A) Replaces lanolin in the skin.
    B) Keeps hands clean.
    C) Inhibits contact of solvent with skin surface.
    D) A cure for chapped, dry hands and feet.

25) Cotton worker's lung, Cotton bract disease, Mill fever, and Brown lung all refer to which of the following terms?

    A) Osteoporosis.
    B) Byssinosis.
    C) Pneumoconiosis.
    D) Occupational bronchitis.

26) A flood destroys your company's operations facility. After the emergency management issues are addressed, your company implements several plans to: Recover critical files and information that had been stored offsite, establish a temporary facility from which operations can be conducted, and inform customers of the situation and how they will be served. These plans are among examples of a comprehensive loss control activity called:

A) Emergency management/emergency response.
B) Situational Awareness.
C) Disaster Recovery/Business Continuity Planning.
D) Business Impact Analysis.

27) The ANSI/ASC Z49.1 is an excellent voluntary consensus standard. The standard sets forth requirements for all aspects of safety and health in the welding environment. It contains information on protection of personnel and the general area, ventilation, fire prevention and protection, and confined spaces. The standard provides advice on the establishment of a "fire watch" during some welding operations. Which of the following statements **best** describes the intent of the ANSI standard concerning the duties of a fire watch?

A) The fire watch must be supervisory personnel caliber and be trained on firefighting, command & control and other emergency procedures.
B) The fire watch should be trained in welding and firefighting to prevent incidents that may go unnoticed by the welder under hood.
C) The fire watch should maintain vigilance for one half hour after welding operations cease.
D) The fire watch is not required for resistance or GMAT welding but is required if heavy cutting using a torch is being attempted.

28) Which of the following lists the three distinct parts of a "means of egress"?

A) Exit access, exit, and exit discharge.
B) Door, passageway, and ramps.
C) Door opening device, door, and exit light.
D) Horizontal exits, stairs, and ramps.

29) A Commercial Motor Vehicle transporting hazardous materials is required to display placards in which of the following locations?
   A) Front, rear and both sides of vehicle.
   B) Front, rear and both sides of hazmat container.
   C) Front, rear, top and both sides of vehicle.
   D) Front, rear, top and both sides of hazmat container.

30) When developing an emergency plan, the first step should be to?
   A) Identify and evaluate the potential disasters.
   B) Assess the potential harm that may be caused.
   C) Evaluate how many company assets are required.
   D) Decide on the chain of command.

31) What is the primary consideration when preparing for a potential disaster?
   A) Selecting the emergency committee.
   B) Identifying a person to be the on-scene commander.
   C) Doing advanced emergency planning.
   D) Having a list of State and Federal directives that you may need.

32) Which of the following correctly identifies a DOT oxidizer placard?
   A) Background yellow, information black.
   B) Lower half black, upper half white.
   C) Lower part white, upper triangle yellow.
   D) Background red, information white/black.

33) Which of the following NFPA standards deals with Fire Extinguishers?
   A) NFPA 10.
   B) NFPA 70.
   C) NFPA 13.
   D) NFPA 30.

34) You discover a deserted chemical dumpsite on company property and observe leaking containers of perchloric acid, ether and other unidentified chemicals. What should you do?
   A) Segregate chemicals by hand.
   B) Call an experienced HAZMAT team.
   C) Call the EOD team.
   D) Remove chemicals to safe storage.

35) Without proper storage, which of the following chemicals exhibit the **most dangerous** properties?
    A) Nitric acid.
    B) Trichloroethylene.
    C) Perchloric acid.
    D) Orthodichlorobenzene.

36) What is the number one consideration in storing chemicals?
    A) Ventilation.
    B) Fire Suppression.
    C) Control of static.
    D) Segregation.

37) When experiencing a natural emergency, emergency preparedness plans usually call for which of the following as the first consideration?
    A) Turn the responsibility over to the authorities for protection of resources.
    B) Safeguard people and abandon systems.
    C) Shutdown processes involving hazardous/toxic materials.
    D) Safeguard both personnel and equipment/processes.

38) Advanced emergency management planning is the best way to minimize potential loss from natural or human caused disasters and accidents. The primary responsibilities of emergency planning must include all the following **except?**
    A) Continuation of operations for the sake of the customers.
    B) Provide for the safety of the employees and the public.
    C) Protect property and the environment.
    D) Establish methods to restore operations to normal as soon as possible.

39) A door latch assembly incorporating a device that releases the latch upon application of a force in the direction of exit travel is the definition of?
    A) Door knob.
    B) Panic hardware.
    C) Secure door guard.
    D) Emergency protection hardware.

40) If you have an emergency response situation and need to set up a command center, always set it up in the:
   A) Cold zone.
   B) Warm zone.
   C) Hot zone.
   D) Outside of all zones.

41) Which of the following is designed to verify if the management system is working, that the emergency management administrative function is adequate and that the lines of communication are operating?
   A) Dry run.
   B) Practice session.
   C) Sandbox exercise.
   D) Tabletop exercise.

42) General guidelines for cleaning up a minor spill of flammable or combustible material, includes all of the following **except?**
   A) Immediately notify OSHA of the spill.
   B) Isolate the spill site from non-required personnel.
   C) Block off the spill are to prevent access.
   D) Remove electric hazards, incompatible chemicals or wastes, physical hazards and sources of ignition.

43) During emergency response planning, you would coordinate will all of the following **except?**
   A) Local Fire Departments.
   B) Local Police Departments.
   C) FEMA.
   D) Local Public Library.

44) The National Incident Management System (NIMS) is the responsibility of the:
   A) Department of State (DOS).
   B) Department of Health and Human Services (DHHS).
   C) Department of Defense (DOD).
   D) Department of Homeland Security (DHS).

45) Which of the following **best** explains the term BLEVE?
  A) Boiling Liquid Expanding Vapor Explosion.
  B) Burning Liquid & Expanding Vapor Explosion.
  C) Boiling Liquid Exacerbated Volume Expansion.
  D) Burning Liquid Elevated Volume Expansion.

46) The one function that will always be filled at every incident, regardless of size is the?
  A) Operations commander.
  B) Incident commander.
  C) Emergency Action coordinator.
  D) Medical staff.

47) What type of fire extinguishing equipment is required for welding operations?
  A) Class A.
  B) Class B.
  C) Class C.
  D) Suitable fire extinguishing equipment.

48) In some industrial occupancies, fire doors are provided to allow compartmentalization of the facility and prevent the spread of fire and smoke. If these doors are equipped with self-closing devices they must be inspected regularly to assure operation. All of the following are valid inspection items **except?**
  A) Check lubrication on guides and bearings.
  B) Check to insure fusible links are painted to prevent rust.
  C) Check binders are not bent, thus obstructing the door.
  D) Check to insure chains or wire ropes have not stretched.

49) During inspections of building sprinklers systems, often the system does not pass the inspections criteria. The leading cause of failure is?
  A) Broken water pipes.
  B) Closed PIV.
  C) Electrical failure.
  D) Lack of pressure.

50) The ASME Boiler and Pressure Vessel Code requires most pressure vessels to have safety devices (i.e. relief valves, fusible plugs, etc.) to adequately protect against overpressure, chemical reaction, or other abnormal conditions. When discharge lines are provided to carry discharge away from safety valves, the area of the discharge pipe should be _____ the area of the valve outlet(s)?
   A) Greater than.
   B) Less than.
   C) Equal to.
   D) Equal to or greater than.

51) The standard requires that all materials stored in tiers be stacked, racked, blocked, interlocked, or otherwise secured to prevent sliding, falling or collapse. Which of the following statements would be the **most correct** concerning the stacking of masonry blocks?
   A) Masonry blocks must not be stacked over 8 feet in height.
   B) Masonry blocks must not be stacked over 10 feet in height.
   C) Masonry blocks stacked higher than 6 feet, must be tapered back one-half block per tier above the 6-foot level.
   D) Masonry blocks stacks must be tapered back 4 inches in every foot of height above the 5-foot level.

52) All materials stored in tiers must be stacked, racked, blocked, interlocked, or otherwise secured to prevent sliding, falling or collapse. Which of the following statements would be correct concerning the stacking of lumber?
   A) Stacked lumber cannot exceed 16 feet.
   B) Lumber must have nails removed or bent over before stacking.
   C) Lumber piles over 12 feet must be handled with fork trucks.
   D) Lumber can be manually stacked no more than 16 feet high.

53) All of the following describe specific requirements concerning potable water on a construction site **except?**
   A) Potable water must be available on the job site immediately following soil compaction tests.
   B) All water containers must be marked and not used for any other purpose.
   C) Drinking from a common cup or from the lid on a water container is not allowed.
   D) If single service cups are provided a dispenser and a disposal receptacle with a lid are required.

54) Which of the following noise exposures exceed the OSHA 1926.52 standards?
   A)   92 dBA for 8 hours.
   B)   110 dBA for 1/4 hour.
   C)   102 dBA for 1 1/2 hours.
   D)   105 dBA for 1 hour.

55) According to OSHA exposure to impulsive or impact noise should **not** exceed _____ peak sound pressure level?
   A)   130 dB.
   B)   115 dB.
   C)   110 dB.
   D)   140 dB.

56) The risk remaining after preventive measures have been taken is called:
   A)   Acceptable risk.
   B)   Tolerable risk.
   C)   Unacceptable risk.
   D)   Residual risk.

57) Follow up inspections are **most likely** used to:
   A) Determine training needs.
   B) Verify compliance.
   C) Discipline workers.
   D) Identify causal factors.

58) Horizontal lifelines with two workers on the same line shall have a minimum breaking strength of:
   A) 13.3 kN.
   B) 5000 lbs.
   C) 22.2 kN.
   D) 10,000 lbs.

59) Accident costs such as loss in earning power, loss of time by supervision, damage to tools and equipment, and cost of training a new worker are also called?
   A)   Direct costs.
   B)   Insured costs.
   C)   Indirect costs.
   D)   Miscellaneous costs.

60) Which of the following **best** describes the use of the Critical Incident Technique method during an incident investigation?
   - A) A method to identify mechanical integrity issues in chemical process equipment.
   - B) An open-ended retrospective method of interviews that identify the critical aspects of an incident.
   - C) A guided discussion as part of pre-emergency planning exercise.
   - D) A sampling of human behaviors through observations.

61) Which is the **best** example of a safety performance benchmark?
   - A) Thorough root cause analysis.
   - B) Incident rate below the industrial average.
   - C) Increased injury trends.
   - D) Employee involvement.

62) You are the Safety Director of a textile plant that has received an OSHA inspection. You were cited for several violations and your citations have been received at the main plant. Which of the following actions is **most correct?**
   - A) You must pay the fine within 15 working days.
   - B) The workers must be allowed to see the citation.
   - C) You must fix the discrepancy within 30 days.
   - D) You must post the citations for at least three days.

63) Medical records maintained under the provisions of 1910.1030 must be retained for what period of time?
   - A) 30 years.
   - B) Duration of employment plus 30 years.
   - C) 5 years.
   - D) Duration of employment plus 5 years.

64) As described in ANSI/ASSE Z10, for an organization's occupational health and safety management system to succeed, top management leadership and which of the following are **most critical?**
   - A) Supervisor accountability.
   - B) Employee participation.
   - C) OHS written policy.
   - D) Sustainable safety observation program.

65) The primary purpose of a safety meeting is:
    A) Provide discipline to workers not following safety rules.
    B) Inform workers of job specific hazards.
    C) Satisfy government regulations.
    D) Company paperwork.

66) If you are going to select a software program to track and monitor your accidents and rates, the **best** option would be:
    A) Data base.
    B) Spread sheet.
    C) Word processing.
    D) Financial management.

67) Which class of employees would you expect to have the greatest potential for accidents?
    A)   New employees.
    B)   Experienced employees.
    C)   Administrative employees.
    D)   Disabled employees.

68) The outside consultant and trainer can be of value as a:
    A)   Change agent.
    B)   Highly skilled first line supervisors.
    C)   Replacement for organizational leadership.
    D)   Decision maker.

69) Which of the following agencies is concerned with pedestrian safety?
    A)   Federal Motor Carrier Safety Administration (FMCSA).
    B)   National Transportation Safety Board (NTSB).
    C)   National Highway Traffic Safety Administration (NHTSA).
    D)   Federal Highway Administration (FHA).

70) Which of the following is an example of an administrative control?
    A)   Standard operating procedure.
    B)   Chemical substitution.
    C)   Personal Protective Equipment.
    D)   Machine Guarding.

71) A description of the company's current performance, and what the company wants to achieve in the future is called a:
  - A) Training evaluation.
  - B) Gap analysis.
  - C) Level four evaluation.
  - D) Proficiency assessment.

72) Which of the following training methods is primarily used to find new, innovative approaches to issues?
  - A) Lecture.
  - B) Brainstorming.
  - C) Case Study.
  - D) Role Playing.

73) Which of the following is first item to be analyzed when implementing a job safety analysis program?
  - A) The order of Jobs according to product flow moving through each department.
  - B) The jobs generating the most complaints from supervisors.
  - C) The jobs contributing to the highest incident rates.
  - D) The jobs exposing the most workers.

74) The company health and safety officer completed a Job Safety Analysis (JSA) for a supervisor's task and forwarded it to the field. Once JSA is received and reviewed with the supervisors in training, it is apparent that there are more hazards to the task than are listed on the JSA. As a trainer, what should you do?
  - A) Send the JSA back to the health and safety officer and do not begin work on the task until the JSA has been revised to reflect status change of hazard.
  - B) Work with the supervisors to understand hazards on JSA and make any corrections to it and send it back to the safety officer.
  - C) Send the JSA back to the health and safety officer.
  - D) Begin training on the task using the information listed on the JSA.

75) When working on scaffold 50 feet high who must approve the scaffold for use?
- A) The Superintendent.
- B) The Supervisor.
- C) The Competent person.
- D) The Engineer.

76) Annual training requirement for a confined space rescue team must include:
- A) PPE training.
- B) Entry Training.
- C) CPR training.
- D) Rescue training.

77) Many safety management training classes provide detailed instruction on the establishment of safety and health committees. Which of the following would **not** be considered a duty of a central safety committee?
- A) Approve purchase requests for safety equipment.
- B) Review design of new plant equipment.
- C) Investigate extra hazardous conditions.
- D) Guide and direct the safety effort.

78) When performing instructor duties for a Health and Safety Training session, it is **most important** to?
- A) Dress for the occasion.
- B) Know what you are talking about.
- C) Use plenty of visual aids.
- D) Use a well-prepared lesson plan.

79) For Construction Health and Safety Training to provide maximum effectiveness, firm training objectives should be established and used. Which of the following requirements of training objectives is the **least important?**
- A) Training objectives should be Reasonable.
- B) Training objectives should be Measurable.
- C) Training objectives should be Obtainable.
- D) Training objectives should be Written.

80) People will model behavior that they view are beneficial; therefore, workers are more prone to follow rules when:
- A) Contractors are seen bypassing rules.
- B) The supervisor follows the rules.
- C) Workers are sometimes disciplined for breaking rules.
- D) They see fellow workers punished when caught breaking rules.

81) Which of the following is of **least importance** when considering an instructor for a Health & Safety Training project in a construction setting?
- A) Knowledge of subject.
- B) Presentation style.
- C) Desire to instruct.
- D) Appearance.

82) Often in safety and health training programmed or instructional learning is used instead of more traditional methods. Which of the following is **most correct** concerning the technique of programmed learning?
- A) Programmed learning is very controversial because it attempts to control the actions of workers.
- B) Programmed learning is confined to computer use only.
- C) Programmed learning is not suitable for complex, complicated endeavors.
- D) Programmed learning is an effective tool for very short study sessions.

83) Safety and health training can involve many different delivery systems and training techniques. Often group methods are used to increase the effectiveness of training and the active participation by students. Which of the following would be the **best** use of the *role-playing* technique?
- A) In human relations training.
- B) For job instruction training in a one-on-one situation.
- C) To illustrate the complexities of a step-by-step detailed industrial task.
- D) For in-depth technical subjects.

84) One technique often used in safety and health training in the industrial environment is the conference method. Which of the following is the **most correct** concerning this important training tool?
   A) Individual knowledge is not particularly important during a conference session.
   B) The conference technique is not particularly suited to problem solving.
   C) The success of the conference technique depends on the ability of the main presenter.
   D) The success of the conference depends almost entirely on the ability of the facilitator.

85) Which of the following fails to describe a requirement of the owners of a hazardous waste site cleanup project, under the provisions of the OSHA 1910.120, site safety and health training program?
   A) Training for all site workers and supervisors.
   B) Training for spill response.
   C) Training for specialists responding to the scene of a spill.
   D) Training on personal protective equipment.

86) One training technique especially useful when dealing with craft employees during safety and health training is the *case study*. Which of the following is the **most correct** concerning a case study?
   A) Case studies must always involve fictitious situations or accidents so that no one group, or person will have hurt feelings.
   B) Case studies should be written and passed out as handouts to be most effective because most craft employees do not have a long attention span.
   C) Case studies are good problem-solving tools.
   D) Case studies involving real situations should only be used if they can be presented by the actual participants/victims.

87) According to NIOSH, to provide the most effective level of safety during confined space entry, which of the following correctly indicates the minimum amount of training necessary?
   A) Recognition of hazardous materials, first-aid training, rescue training and orientation on self-contained breathing apparatus.
   B) Confined space hazard recognition training, training for testing hazardous atmospheres, training on rescue procedures, training on PPE and advanced first-aid training.
   C) Confined space hazard recognition training, training for testing hazardous atmospheres, training on rescue procedures, training on PPE and first-aid training.
   D) Recognition of hazardous materials, advanced first-aid training, training on rescue procedures, and in-depth training on the use of self-contained breathing equipment.

88) Who must be trained for working on a scaffold?
   A) All workers.
   B) Competent persons.
   C) Workers who assemble or dismantle scaffolds.
   D) Workers above 10 feet.

89) Behavior is most influenced by:
   A) Activators.
   B) Consequences.
   C) Discipline.
   D) Feedback.

90) The U.S. OSHA standard 1910.120, Hazardous Waste Operations and Emergency Response, requires training for waste site workers, occasional workers, and site supervisors. Which of the following **best** describes the training required for the general hazardous waste site worker?
   A) 40 hours of training on-site, with at least 2 days field experience under a trained supervisor.
   B) 24 hours training on-site, and two days hands-on.
   C) 24 hours training off-site, one day hands-on.
   D) 40 hours of training off-site, with at least 3 days field experience under a trained supervisor.

91) Which of the following is the **most often recommended** fundamental safety training for construction workers?
   A) First Aid, Supervisors Safety, and Welding.
   B) Welding, Fork truck Training, and Back-Care.
   C) Fire Extinguisher Training, First Aid, and Contingency.
   D) Contingency, First Aid and Vehicle Operations.

92) When is the **least effective** time to present a safety training session?
   A) After an accident.
   B) After the company announces it is downsizing.
   C) After the monthly accident data shows an increase in the incident rate.
   D) After a plant explosion.

93) All of the following substances are excluded from the OSHA Hazard Communication Standard labeling requirements **except?**
   A) Cosmetics.
   B) Pesticides.
   C) Wood products including wood dust.
   D) Hazardous waste.

94) Training is primarily focused on behavior change. In education, the focus is on information about something that may or may not be used on the job. In training, the focus is also on how to do something properly and how to apply the new information and skills on the job. The benefits of safety and health training include all the following **except?**
   A) Improved performance.
   B) Fewer accidents.
   C) Reduced costs.
   D) Attitude adjustment.

95) Which of the following is **not** considered to be an effective training method?
   A) Demonstration.
   B) Technical speech.
   C) Guided discussion.
   D) Individualized instruction.

96) Which of the following is a primary desirable attribute of a safety training instructor?

    A) Always uses an overhead projector.

    B) Covers the course content and adds many war stories.

    C) Enhances the presentation with many scientific and technical terms.

    D) Covers the quantity of material as outlined by the course objectives.

97) When you develop the tests and evaluations for your training program, you should use all of the following guidelines **except?**

    A) Test items must be reliable.

    B) Evaluations are norm-referenced.

    C) Each test item must have criterion-related validity.

    D) The evaluation tool should be developed before the training begins.

98) Which of the following training methods allows for the **least** amount of student-instructor interaction?

    A) Lecture.

    B) Role playing.

    C) Case study.

    D) Facilitated discussion.

99) Which of the following is **not** a required training item under the OSHA Hazard Communication Standard?

    A) Work area operations containing hazardous chemicals.

    B) Location of hazardous chemical list & SDS.

    C) Plant emergency evacuation plan.

    D) Details of the labeling system.

100) Which of the following is the **most correct** concerning the OSHA Hazard Communication requirement for the maintenance of worker training records?

    A) Training records must be maintained by the employee.

    B) Training records must be maintained by the employer.

    C) Training records must be maintained at the worksite.

    D) There is no requirement in OSHA to maintain a worker's training record.

Self-Assessment Exam One Answers

1). Answer D:

OSHA 3151-12R 2004 Personal Protective Equipment states that safety footwear must meet ANSI minimum compression and impact performance standards in ANSI Z41 (American National Standard for Personal Protection-Protective Footwear) All ANSI-approved footwear has a protective toe and offers impact and compression protection. But the type and amount of protection is not always the same. Different footwear protects in different ways. Foot and leg protection choices include the following:

- Leggings protect the lower legs and feet from heat hazards such as molten metal or welding sparks. Safety snaps allow leggings to be removed quickly.
- Metatarsal guards protect the instep area from impact and compression. Made of aluminum, steel, fiber or plastic, these guards may be strapped to the outside of shoes.
- Toe guards fit over the toes of regular shoes to protect the toes from impact and compression hazards. They may be made of steel, aluminum or plastic.
- Combination foot and shin guards protect the lower legs and feet, and may be used in combination with toe guards when greater protection is needed.
- Safety shoes have impact-resistant toes and heat-resistant soles that protect the feet against hot work surfaces common in roofing, paving and hot metal industries. The metal insoles of some safety shoes protect against puncture wounds. Safety shoes may also be designed to be electrically conductive to prevent the buildup of static electricity in areas with the potential for explosive atmospheres or nonconductive to protect employees from workplace electrical hazards.

2). Answer B:

Fibrosis is a condition in which the lung becomes scarred and inflexible, making the lung unable to expand and contract.

3). Answer C:

All respirators can be placed in two categories:

- air-purifying
- air-supplying

4). Answer B:

A combination of goggles vented or non-vented and a face shield provides the *best* protection from the damaging effects of heavy metal grinding. Face shields are also required for any splashing hazard.

5). Answer B:

Job redesign by moving the maintenance work station outside of the hazard area to eliminate the exposure risk to the robot hazards while performing duties at the work station. De-energizing or Lock out of the robot, light curtains, enclosures are an example of an engineering control. The lock out procedure and training are administrative controls.

6). Answer A:

Assigned Protection Factor (APF) means the workplace level of respiratory protection that a respirator or class of respirators is expected to provide to employees when the employer implements a continuing, effective respiratory protection program as specified by this section.

Assigned Protection Factors					
Type of Respirator	Quarter mask	Half mask	Full facepiece	Helmet/Hood	Loose-fitting facepiece
1. Air-Purifying Respirator	5	10	50	—	—
2. Powered Air-Purifying	—	50	1,000	25/1,000	25
Supplied-Air Respirator (SAR) or Airline Respirator					
• Demand mode	—	10	50	— 25/1,000	— 25
• Continuous flow mode	—	50	1,000	—	—
• Pressure-demand or other positive-pressure mode	—	50	1,000		
Self-Contained Breathing Apparatus (SCBA)					
• Demand mode	—	10	50	50	—
• Pressure-demand or other positive- pressure mode	—	—	10,000	10,000	—
OSHA 3352-02 2009 Assigned Protection Factors for the Revised Respiratory					

7). Answer C:

If a tagout system is used it must provide full employee protection. This means that the employer must demonstrate that the tagout system will provide a level of safety equivalent to that obtained by using a lockout program. Generally this means the removal of an actuating device e.g.: the handle on a valve, the removal of a fuse or circuit switch etc.

8). Answer C:

GTAW stands for Gas Tungsten Arc-Welding, which is a process that joins metals by heating them with an arc between a tungsten electrode and the work, shielding is obtained from a gas mixture. The process is often called TIG welding. Because of the inherent safety and health hazards involved in the welding process the CHST examination may have several questions on the different processes and the hazards associated with each.

9). Answer D:

The question does not tell us anything about the atmosphere in the confined space, respirators may not even be required. Without any other detail one must assume that the conditions within the confined space are IDLH and oxygen deficient, in which case the best and safest choice is the airline with an escape supply.

10). Answer A:

Only the gas mask is an air purifying type of respirator the others all are air supplying.

11). Answer C:

The inertia of an object in motion increases when there is an increase or decrease in speed. This change in inertia causes great increases in stress forces placed on the rigging. As a load line starts to move, sudden accelerations can cause as much as twice the stress on the rigging as the actual load. This is why most rigging or hoisting instructions contain warnings or cautions about applying lifting forces in a slow and smooth manner.

12). Answer C:

Rubber gloves, and other rubber goods, are often used for protection against contact with high voltage conductors. There are several classes of gloves however most require leather outer gloves for protection. Shown below is a short instruction sheet included with rubber gloves from a major distributor.

CLASS 00 INSULATING RUBBER GLOVES

Leather protectors should always be used and worn over your insulating gloves. They provide mechanical protection for rubber insulating gloves only and when used alone do not provide any protection against serious injury, death, or other potential dangers from electrical shocks or burns. The protection should be inspected at the same time rubber gloves are inspected. Look for metal particles, imbedded wire, abrasive materials or any substance that could cause puncture, abrasion, contamination or deterioration. To maintain an adequate flashover distance between the top of the protector and bead of the rubber glove, the protector cuff should bend at least one inch below the bead.

Where the finger dexterity necessary to manipulate small equipment and parts requires use of Class 00 gloves without leather protectors, extra care must be taken by the user to prevent puncture, abrasion and other damage to the gloves. To assure their continued integrity, Class 00 gloves used under these conditions should be inspected more frequently than when used with leather protectors.

Class 00 used in this example is the lowest class of protection (500 volts). Additional information is contained in the ANSI J6 series standards and in the ASTM F496 specification for in-service care of gloves and sleeves. Generally, in-service gloves must be tested at intervals not to exceed 6 months and a record of test voltages and dates must be kept. The last date of testing must be marked on the glove itself and it must be kept in a container designed for and used exclusively for gloves or rubber goods.

13). Answer B:

When setting up a straight ladder the base should be one-fourth the ladder length from the vertical plane of the top support.

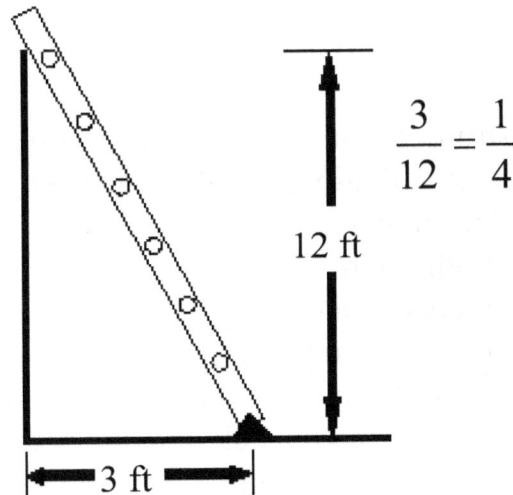

$$\frac{3}{12} = \frac{1}{4}$$

12 ft

3 ft

14). Answer B:

Direct reading instrumentation is a very broad category and ranges from detector tubes to portable gas chromatographs that are capable of detecting just about every chemical one could encounter. Additionally, direct reading instrumentation can be very accurate or, in the case of detector tubes, not so accurate. However, direct reading instrumentation does suffer from one common ailment, almost all of these instruments suffer from interference by other contaminates.

15). Answer D:

Based on the statement in the question that there were no changes in plant operations we feel the best course of action would be to stop monitoring and recalibrate the instrumentation. The reading of 65 ppm is not life threatening and recalibration should be able to be accomplished in fresh air in a very short time.

16) Answer A:

According to ANSI A14.1, *Safety Requirements for Portable Wood Ladders*, "Ladders may be coated with a suitable protective material." The theory is that any cracks, splits, chips, rot or compression failures can be spotted through an opaque or clear finish such as varnish, lacquer or shellac.

17) Answer D:

Geiger-Muller instruments are widely used in survey work and are extremely sensitive to radiation. A discrimination shield is used and when open will admit both gamma and beta emissions. When closed gamma radiation is admitted. The "Cutie pie" is perhaps one of the most widely used instruments available for radiological survey work. They are intended to measure only X-ray and gamma radiation, although some have thin "end-windows" which also allow beta particles measurement. The condenser R-meters are very reliable and accurate instruments for measuring exposures of X and gamma rays. Because of the condenser R-meters great precision, it is frequently used as a secondary standard. There is no known device called a "Scatter Absorber".

18) Answer C:

OSHA 1926.451 requires all scaffolds and their components to be capable of supporting without failure at least 4 times the maximum intended load. Safety factor is defined as:

$$\frac{\text{Breaking strength}}{\text{Maximum load}} = \text{Safety Factor}$$

Or stated another way, with a safety factor of four the maximum allowable load will never be greater than 25% of the load it takes to cause the scaffold to fail. Safety factors are developed to allow for greater than anticipated:

- Loads (extra men, equipment etc.)
- Wind loading
- Faulty and defective equipment
- Poor scaffold design

1926.451(f)(5) Scaffolds shall not be moved horizontally while employees are on them, unless they have been designed by a registered professional engineer specifically for such movement

19) Answer C:

OSHA requires that any scaffold that exceeds a platform height to smallest base dimension of four be equipped with outriggers to increase the base dimension or they can be guyed or otherwise tied down. However, be careful the CHST examination is based on Federal OSHA, requirements in both California and Ohio are more stringent.

20) Answer D:

OSHA at 1926.451 provides specific guidance concerning scaffolding. A good review of this section is in order prior to taking the CHST examination. Selection "A" is correct, scaffold planking must be at least 1500 psi fiber (Stress Grade) scaffold grade lumber. This 1500 psi fiber refers to the strength of the lumber in bending. Selection "B" is correct. Selection "C" is also correct, OSHA offers this chart from which to select spans.

MATERIAL					
	Full thickness undressed lumber			Nominal Thickness Lumber	
Working load (psf)	25	50	75	25	50
Permissible span (ft)	10	8	6	8	6

Selection "D" is obviously incorrect, the sill and base plate is a very important part of the overall scaffold foundation. Often the base plate cannot adequately distribute the high loads from the scaffold, in this case a timber sill is required. The sill provides a friction surface and spreads loads over a larger area than the base plate. Sills are most often wood, but come in many different sizes depending on the loads involved. Often a 2 × 10 wood sill is used, it should be continuous and should be centered under the leg and provide a bearing surface for at least two legs. Obviously, bricks or cement blocks are just not adequate and are prohibited by OSHA.

21) Answer C:

Substances that are capable of damaging the liver are called ***hepatotoxins.***

22) Answer B:

Additive Effect (2 + 2 = 4) Some toxic chemicals add their effects together in producing a biological effect. In this case the effect is the same as being exposed to double the dose of either chemical alone. Example: acetaminophen and ibuprofen.

Synergistic Effect (2 + 2 = 6) Synergism is the exposure to two different toxic chemicals that produce a more severe effect than simply doubling the dose of either one alone. An example is isopropyl alcohol and chloroform. The alcohol ties up the enzymes that would normally break down chloroform.

Potentiation (0 + 2 = 10) In some cases a chemical without any known toxic effect may act together with a known toxic substance to make the toxic substance even more potent and thus more dangerous. Ethanol (ethyl alcohol) and chloroform together affect the liver in just such a manner.

Antagonism (4 + 6 = 8) The interaction of two toxic chemicals may be such that the effect produced is actually less than would be expected. Phenobarbital and benzopyrene together is an example. The Phenobarbital increases the enzyme activity that detoxifies the benzopyrene.

23) Answer C:

Hepatitis B Virus (HBV). The hepatitis B virus infects the liver. In some individuals, HBV develops into serious or fatal problems, such as cirrhosis, liver cancer, or chronic liver disease. Some people have no problems or symptoms yet become carriers of the virus. HBV is more common and is a much hardier virus than HIV; it can exist on a surface outside the body for up to thirty days. For this reason, it poses a greater hazard to an exposed individual. Human Immunodeficiency Virus (HIV). Hepatitis A Virus (HAV). Hepatitis C Virus (HCV).

24) Answer C:

Protective creams sometimes called "Barrier" creams serve to inhibit contact with solvents in the work place. The use of protective creams is very controversial, however most of the current Safety and Health literature indicates, when used properly, these creams are useful. The cream must be used correctly to be effective which means it must be applied on clean skin at the beginning of the work shift, removed at lunch, reapplied after lunch, again in the afternoon, and removed at the close of the work shift.

25)   Answer B:

Byssinosis, also called "brown lung disease" or "Monday fever", is an occupational lung disease caused by exposure to cotton dust in inadequately ventilated working environments. Byssinosis commonly occurs in workers who are employed in yarn and fabric manufacture industries. It is not thought that the cotton dust directly causes the disease, and some believe that the causative agents are endotoxins that come from the cell walls of gram negative bacteria that grow on the cotton. Although bacterial endotoxin is a likely cause, the absence of similar symptoms in workers in other industries exposed to endotoxins makes this uncertain.

26)   Answer C:

According to Risk Analysis and the Security Survey, 3rd Edition, business continuity planning is a key part of a loss control program. Such plans should include recovering corporate information, setting up operations, and financing temporary operations until a new facility can be commissioned. Depending upon the risk of a natural disaster, some companies purchase business interruption insurance to help finance operations.

27)   Answer C:

Several organizations and standards offer suggestions on establishment of a "fire watch" for welding and cutting operations including ANSI Z49.1, OSHA 1910.252 and NFPA 51B etc. OSHA has this to say concerning fire watchers: "Fire watchers shall have fire extinguishing equipment readily available and be trained on its use. They shall be familiar with facilities for sounding an alarm in the event of a fire. They shall watch for fires in all exposed areas, try to extinguish them only when obviously within the capacity of the equipment available, or otherwise sound the alarm. A fire watch shall be maintained for at least one half hour after completion of welding or cutting operations to detect and extinguish possible smoldering fires".

28) Answer A:

NFPA 101, Life Safety Code, states, "A means of egress is a continuous and unobstructed way of exit travel from any point in a building or structure to a public way and consists of three separate and distinct parts: (a) the exit access, (b) the exit, and (c) the exit discharge. A means of egress comprises the vertical and horizontal travel and shall include intervening room spaces, doorways, hallways, corridors, passageways, balconies, ramps, stairs, enclosures, lobbies, escalators, horizontal exits, courts, and yards. It does not include elevators.

29) Answer A:

According to 49 CFR 172.504, placards should be attached as you load and before you drive the vehicle. The placards must appear on both sides and ends of the vehicle. Each placard must be

- easily seen from the direction it faces
- placed so the words or numbers are level and read from left to right
- at least three inches from other markings.

30) Answer A:

Although all the answers need to be addressed during the planning process, according to the NSC, "Before an organization initiates an emergency plan, it should identify and evaluate the potential disasters that might occur". During the follow on of this process, you may have to develop mutual aid agreement with other companies or agencies in order to mitigate the emergencies or disasters.

31) Answer C:

According to the NSC, "advanced emergency management planning is the best way to minimize potential loss from natural or human caused disasters or accidents."

32) Answer A because:

Answer B is the color for a corrosive sign or placard.
Answer C is the color for a radioactive sign or placard.
Answer D is the color for a combustible sign or placard.

33) Answer A:

NFPA 10 is the Standard for Portable Fire Extinguishers. Remember that if you expect your employees to use portable fire extinguishers, they must be trained.

34) Answer B:

As you are dealing with some potentially unstable chemicals, you should call in experts.

35) Answer C:

Perchloric acid with age can become unstable. One indication is crystal growth around the lid. It becomes very shock sensitive and can readily explode. Denatured (old) Ether exhibits the same hazard.

36) Answer D:

The first principle of good storage practice for chemicals is segregation, including separation from other materials in storage, from processing and handling operations and from incompatible materials.

1926.152(b) "Indoor storage of flammable and combustible liquids.": No more than 25 gallons of flammable or combustible liquids shall be stored in a room outside of an approved storage cabinet. Quantities of flammable and combustible liquid in excess of 25 gallons shall be stored in an acceptable or approved cabinet meeting the following requirements: Acceptable wooden storage cabinets shall be constructed in the following manner, or equivalent: The bottom, sides, and top shall be constructed of an exterior grade of plywood at least 1 inch in thickness, which shall not break down or delaminate under standard fire test conditions. All joints shall be rabbeted and shall be fastened in two directions with flathead wood screws. When more than one door is used, there shall be a rabbeted overlap of not less than 1 inch. Steel hinges shall be mounted in such a manner as to not lose their holding capacity due to loosening or burning out of the screws when subjected to fire. Such cabinets shall be painted inside and out with fire retardant paint. Approved metal storage cabinets will be acceptable. Cabinets shall be labeled in conspicuous lettering, "Flammable-Keep Fire Away." Not more than 60 gallons of flammable or 120 gallons of combustible liquids shall be stored in any one storage cabinet. Not more than three such cabinets may be located in a single storage area. Quantities in excess of this shall be stored in an inside storage room.

37) Answer D:

When planning for an emergency one must consider the protection of all resources. Naturally the saving of life must come first, however protection of processes and equipment is also of utmost concern. Should the decision be made to abandon hazardous processes, an additional disaster could be created.

38) Answer A:

According to the National Safety Council, advanced emergency management planning should include the following and they should be ranked as they are sequenced.

1). provide for the safety of the employees and the public
2). protect property and the environment
3). establish methods to restore operations to normal as soon as possible

39) Answer B:

According to the Life Safety Code, this is the definition of panic hardware or fire exit hardware and should be used on doors that need to be secured.

40) Answer A:

Always position the command center or command post in the area of least exposure or in the cold zone.

41) Answer D:

This is the definition of a table top exercise.

42) Answer A:

You are not required to notify OSHA for a minor spill, however you need to isolate the area for cleanup and remove all hazards, including ignition sources, especially if the spill is flammable.

43) Answer D:

Disaster plans should be drawn up in advance and include, neighboring companies, community agencies, including police and fire departments, industry and medical agencies and governmental agencies.

44) Answer D because

The *National Incident Management System (NIMS)*, is the responsibility of the Department of Homeland Security (DHS). It provides a consistent template for managing incidents is a companion document to the National Response Framework and provides standard command and management structures that apply to response activities. This system provides a consistent, nationwide template to enable Federal, State, tribal, and local governments, the private sector, and Non-governmental Organizations (NGOs) to work together to prepare for, prevent, respond to, recover from, and mitigate the effects of incidents, regardless of cause, size, location, or complexity. This consistency provides the foundation for utilization of the NIMS for all incidents, ranging from daily occurrences to incidents requiring a coordinated Federal response.

45) Answer A:

The term BLEVE is the acronym for a Boiling Liquid Expanding Vapor Explosion, which is a major container rupture due to a form of pressure release explosion. This can be caused from external heating such as an adjacent container fire. For this reason, the fire attack scenario of a tank fire would include hose streams directed on adjacent containers as well as the burning tank.

46) Answer B:

According to the NSC, the one function that will always be filled at every incident, regardless of size is the incident commander. For small operations, the most likely incident commander will be the Fire Chief, because of the greater experience, more equipment involved and more training than the facility staff.

47)   Answer D:

1910.252(a)(2)(ii): Fire extinguishers. Suitable fire extinguishing equipment shall be maintained in a state of readiness for instant use. Such equipment may consist of pails of water, buckets of sand, hose or portable extinguishers depending upon the nature and quantity of the combustible material exposed. Class C might be needed if the welding equipment catches on fire. Also Class D might be needed for a metal fire.

48)   Answer B:

Fusible lead links should not be painted because the paint affects the temperature at which the links will melt. The best source for data on testing and certifying or approving fire-rated doors is Factory Mutual Global (FM Global).

49)   Answer B:

The most common cause of building sprinkler system failure is that someone has closed the post-indicator valve (PIV) and failed to reopen it.

An annual inspection is required for hanger bracing, pipe and fitting, sprinklers and fire department connections.

50)   Answer D:

According to ASME B31 series, *Pressure Piping*, sectional areas of a discharge pipe shall not be less than the full area of the valve outlets discharging there into and the discharge pipe shall be as short as possible and so arranged as to avoid undue stresses on the valve or valves. It is recommended that individual discharge lines be used for each valve, but if two or more valves are combined, the discharge piping shall be designed with sufficient flow area to prevent blowout of steam or other fluids.

51)   Answer C:

According to OSHA at 1926.250(b)(7) "When masonry blocks are stacked higher than 6 feet, the stack shall be tapered back one-half block per tier above the 6-foot level".

52) Answer D:

According to OSHA at 1926.250(b)(8) Lumber:

- Used lumber shall have all nails withdrawn before stacking
- Lumber shall be stacked on level and solidly supported sills
- Lumber shall be so stacked as to be stable and self-supporting
- Lumber piles shall not exceed 20 feet in height provided that lumber to be handled manually shall not be stacked more than 16 feet high

53) Answer A:

Field sanitation is a major concern on a construction site, of importance is the subject of drinking water. Accordingly, the rules concerning sanitation and drinking water are strict in the OSHA Standards. OSHA requires all job sites have an adequate supply of potable water. This includes the "dirt work" phase of construction through installation of sanitary facilities. OSHA 1926.51 states:

- "An adequate supply of potable water shall be provided in all places of employment.
- Portable containers used to dispense drinking water shall be capable of being tightly closed, and equipped with a tap. Water shall not be dipped from containers.
- Any container used to distribute drinking water shall be clearly marked as to the nature of its contents and not be used for any other purpose.
- The common drinking cup is prohibited.
- Where single service cups (to be used but once) are supplied, both sanitary container for the unused cups and a receptacle for disposing of the used cups shall be provided."

54) Answer A:

OSHA at 1926.52 allows the following permissible noise exposures.

55) Answer D:

OSHA at 1910.95 and 1926.52 requires exposure to impulsive or impact noise to be limited to 140 dB peak sound pressure level.

56) Answer D:

Residual risk is defined as the risk remaining after preventive measures have been taken. No matter how effective the preventive actions, residual risk will always be present if a facility or operation continues to exist.

57) Answer B:

The primary purpose of follow-up inspections is to verify that corrective action has been successfully implemented. In the case of OSHA inspections, follow-up or abatement verification inspections are used to verify compliance.

58) Answer D:

29 CFR 1926.502 states that Horizontal lifelines shall be designed, installed, and used, under the supervision of a qualified person, as part of a complete personal fall arrest system, which maintains a safety factor of at least two. Lanyards and vertical lifelines shall have a minimum breaking strength of 5,000 pounds (22.2 kN). Except as provided in paragraph (d)(10)(ii) of this section, when vertical lifelines are used, each employee shall be attached to a separate lifeline. During the construction of elevator shafts, two employees may be attached to the same lifeline in the hoistway, provided both employees are working atop a false car that is equipped with guardrails; the strength of the lifeline is 10,000 pounds [5,000 pounds per employee attached] (44.4 kN); and all other criteria specified in this paragraph for lifelines have been met.

59) Answer C:

Accident costs such as loss in earning power, loss of time by supervision, damage to tools and equipment, and cost of training a new worker are also called indirect costs.

60) Answer B:

The **Critical Incident Technique** (or **CIT**) is a set of procedures used for collecting first hand observations of human behavior that have critical significance and meet methodically defined criteria. A critical incident can be described as one that makes a significant contribution—either positively or negatively—to an activity or phenomenon and to understand the relationship between competencies and reasons for accidents. Critical incidents can be gathered in various ways, but typically respondents are asked to tell a story about an experience they have had. Through the use of the critical incident technique one may collect specific and significant behavioral facts, providing a sound basis for making inferences as to requirements for measures of typical performance (criteria), measures of proficiency (standard samples), training, selection and classification, job design, operating procedures, equipment design, motivation and leadership (attitudes), and individual behavior. Critical incidents can be gathered in various ways, but typically respondents are asked to tell a story about an experience they have had. CIT is a flexible method that usually relies on five major areas. The first is determining and reviewing the incident, then fact-finding, which involves collecting the details of the incident from the participants. When all of the facts are collected, the next step is to identify the issues. Afterwards a decision can be made on how to resolve the issues based on various possible solutions. The final and most important aspect is the evaluation, which will determine if the solution that was selected will solve the root cause of the situation and will cause no further problems.

61) Answer B:

According to author Dan Peterson in *Safety by Objectives*, a safety performance benchmark is similar to a goal. A benchmark is based on research conducted on other similar organizations and applied to one's own organization.

62) Answer D:

You are required by OSHA to post the citation at or near the location of the violation for three days or until corrected whichever is longer.

63) Answer B:

Medical records maintained under the provisions of 1910.1030, Bloodborne Pathogens, must be retained for the duration of employment plus 30 years.

64)   Answer B:

According to *ANSI/ASSE Z10 standard*, top management leadership and employee participation are the main divisions in the scope of this standard.

65)   Answer B:

There are several purposes and outcomes of safety meetings. The major purpose is to inform workers of job specific hazards.

66)   Answer B:

A spreadsheet is a computer program that enables you to develop and perform all sorts of calculations between the text and values stored in the document. Most spreadsheets include charting and limited database capabilities.

67)   Answer A:

According to the NSC, although statistical data differ, it is generally agreed that new employees are significantly more prone to work-related accidents.

68)   Answer A:

The outside consultant and trainer can be a particular value as a change agent in an environment of low trust when first line supervisors have marginally low skills, there are pockets of turf that prevent departments from cooperating there is poor alignment across levels of management concerning values that support good safety training. The trainee should always have questions pertinent to the subject matter regardless of the trainer.

69)   Answer D:

The Federal Motor Carrier Safety Administration (FMCSA) was established to reduce crashes, injuries, and fatalities involving large trucks and buses. The Federal Motor Carrier Safety Administration (FMCSA) may prohibit a state from issuing, renewing, transferring, or upgrading CDLs if the agency determined the state is in substantial noncompliance with the CDL licensing and sanctioning requirements.

The National Transportation Safety Board (NTSB) oversees safety in the many branches of the Department of Transportation and reports on all aircraft accidents and major surface accidents. The National Highway Traffic Safety Administration (NHTSA) has responsibility for vehicle safety. It has published over 400 standards on vehicles and vehicle systems. The Federal Highway Administration (FHA) is concerned with administering the highway construction budget and has safety responsibility only for roadways, traffic control devices and pedestrian safety.

70) Answer A:

Administrative controls may include: policy, work rules, Standard Operating Procedures (SOPs), Conduct JSAs, job rotation, inspections, training, coaching and mentoring.

71) Answer B:

A gap analysis can be used to help achieve certain goals. The difference between these two items is the gap. The analysis includes specific action steps the company must complete to close this gap and achieve its goals. Training gap analysis is a measurement of the level of skills possessed by employees at any given moment in relation to the optimal level of skills they need for optimal productivity. The reason for an assessment of a training gap is to help organizations discover inconsistencies within the employee output they currently have. Gaining an idea of what type of skills their employees have will help these organizations know how to tackle the issue of further training for workers. Any company with employees who do not have the highest level of skills to perform their required duties will find themselves at a disadvantage. This aspect is of great importance in a competitive market where every company is trying to outdo the other in every area, including productivity. The methods for initiating and conducting a training gap analysis vary among organizations. Smaller companies with only a few employees may conduct a training gap assessment simply by observing their employees. Organizations generally have the discretion to decide at what times to initiate a training gap analysis. This may be done when there is a safety concern, lag in production or if the qualities of products or services fall below the expected levels. When safety observations indicate a raised level of at risk behavior or an increase in injuries, management may decide to conduct a training gap analysis as part of the investigation into the reasons for the performance discrepancy.

72) Answer B:

Brainstorming is a technique of group interactions that encourages each participant to present ideas on a specific issue. The method is normally used to find new, innovative approaches to issues. There are four ground rules:

- Ideas presented are not criticized.
- Freewheeling creative thinking and building on ideas are positively reinforced.
- As many ideas as possible should be presented quickly.
- Combining several ideas or improving suggestions is encouraged.

Brainstorming			
Advantages	Limitations	Uses	Types of Objectives
Interactive Relevant Creative Can be entertaining.	Time consuming. Requires skilled facilitator	Problem solving Trouble shoot Enhanced by pictures/media.	Best for knowledge-level objectives, Problem Solving

73) Answer C:

In the NSC Accident Prevention Manual for Business and Industry: Administration and Programs. 12th Edition, the jobs selected for job safety analyses should not be selected at random. The order of analysis should be guided by the following factors.

- Frequency of incidents
- Rate of disabling injuries
- Severity potential
- New jobs

74) Answer B:

Work with the supervisors to update the JSA as they have intimate knowledge of the job and should be active participants in the training.

Read and understand the hazards on the JSA and make any corrections to it prior to use. The revised version should be sent to the company safety officer.

75) Answer C:

1926.451(a)(3) No scaffold shall be erected, moved, dismantled, or altered except under the supervision of competent persons.

1926.451(b)(16) All wood pole scaffolds 60 feet or less in height shall be constructed and erected in accordance with Tables L-4 to 10. If they are over 60 feet in height, they shall be designed by a qualified engineer competent in this field, and it shall be constructed and erected in accordance with such design.

1926.451(c)(4) and (5) Tube and coupler scaffolds shall be limited in heights and working levels to those permitted in Tables L- 10, 11, and 12. Drawings and specifications of all tube and coupler scaffolds above the limitations in Tables L- 10, 11, and 12 shall be designed by a qualified engineer competent in this field. All tube and coupler scaffolds shall be constructed and erected to support four times the maximum intended loads, as set forth in Tables L- 10, 11, and 12, or as set forth in specifications by a licensed professional engineer competent in this field.

1926.451(d)(9) Drawings and specifications for all frame scaffolds over 125 feet in height above base plates shall be designed by a registered professional engineer.

1926.451(g)(3) Unless outrigger scaffolds are designed by a registered professional engineer competent in this field, they shall be constructed and erected in accordance with Table L-13. Outrigger scaffolds, designed by a registered professional engineer, and constructed and erected in accordance with such design.

76) Answer D:

According to OSHA 1910.146(k)(2) An employer whose employees have been designated to provide permit space rescue and emergency services shall take the following measures:

- Provide affected employees with the personal protective equipment (PPE) needed to conduct permit space rescues safely and train affected employees so they are proficient in the use of that PPE, at no cost to those employees;

- Train affected employees to perform assigned rescue duties. The employer must ensure that such employees successfully complete the training required to establish proficiency as an authorized entrant, as provided by paragraphs (g) and (h) of this section;
- Train affected employees in basic first-aid and cardiopulmonary resuscitation (CPR). The employer shall ensure that at least one member of the rescue team or service holding a current certification in first aid and CPR is available; and
- Ensure that affected employees practice making permit space rescues at least once every 12 months, by means of simulated rescue operations in which they remove dummies, manikins, or actual persons from the actual permit spaces or from representative permit spaces. Representative permit spaces shall, with respect to opening size, configuration, and accessibility, simulate the types of permit spaces from which rescue is to be performed.

77) Answer A:

Safety Committees to be effective should not be concerned with the day-to-day activities of the safety program within the company...that is, they should not purchase safety equipment, or investigate minor hazards or accidents. They should be responsible for direction of the overall safety effort and provide guidance for the various program elements.

78) Answer D:

The use of a lesson plan will provide standardization to a presentation and avoid omission of essential material. The lesson plan also helps the instructor conduct the class according to a timetable and should provide for student participation or involvement.

79) Answer D:

Training objectives should above all be reasonable, measurable and obtainable. It is very desirable, but not imperative that the objectives and goals for any program to be written, so as not to be misplaced or relegated to a low priority.

80) Answer B:

Workers are more likely to follow rules when the supervisor leads by example and follow the rules

81) Answer D:

There are many attributes that complement a successful trainer or educator. Some of these are:

- Experience
- Honesty
- Knowledge of subject
- Appearance
- Desire to instruct
- Ability to communicate
- Presentation style
- Sensitivity to people

Some of these attributes are more important than others. The motivation of the students and their level of sophistication will determine to a great extent which attribute is the most important. In a construction setting appearance is generally considered to be of lesser importance than the desire to instruct, knowledge of subject and presentation style. This is not to say appearance is not important, just that it is of lesser impact on the learning process.

82) Answer D:

Programmed or instructional learning is an excellent tool for learning just about anything. However, the development of programmed or instructional learning text books or computer programs is very expensive in both time and money. The newer programmed or instructional learning techniques involve interactive computer products. These products combine the features of video and small computers to produce a product that leads the student step-by-step through the learning process. The older instructional learning methods use the text book approach that is presented in a series of numbered pages called *frames*, each frame consists of three parts:

- explanation of a concept
- questions based on the concept
- a "book" answer to the concept

Should the student answer the question incorrectly, some programmed lessons lead the student to another more detailed explanation of the concept.   A programmed text or computer program is extremely useful to persons who must study for short periods of time due to hectic schedules. An additional advantage of this system is that you can study very effectively when you are tired or preoccupied because it provides a lot of repetition and forces you to stay focused. Unlike conventional learning programs, programmed learning is excellent for studying when you have a spare moment. Short periods spent on programmed learning are just as effective as longer sessions.

83)   **Answer A:**

Role playing is ideally suited for human relations education or training. It allows the students to become participants in a "drama" or "play" that depicts the interaction of humans during stressful or error provocative situations. The technique is not suited for problem solving or technical training.

84)   **Answer D:**

One of the most valuable group techniques is the conference method. The strength of the conference method is in the individual knowledge and experience of the participants. The number of members should be kept small to allow maximum exchange of ideas. The establishment of goals and objectives is crucial to the success of this method. But more than anything else, this teaching method hinges on the capability of the facilitator or instructor. The facilitator logs the objectives and keeps the information and opinions flowing during sessions. After the conference, the facilitator distributes recommendations and informs members of actions taken as a result. Shortfalls associated with this method is the facilitator ensuring that the conference does not become a bull session and if management does not follow up on the recommendations, then the group will not support future efforts.

85)   **Answer C:**

OSHA 1910.120 requires an extensive safety and health plan that includes a safety and health training plan. There are extensive requirements outlined in the HAZWOPER standard on the various levels and complexity of training. Training for responding specialists, such as Hazmat teams, is required but generally the responsibility for this training would fall upon their employer, rather than the owner of the clean-up contract.

86) Answer C:

The case study is an especially effective technique for safety and health training, since it often illustrates the multi-causal aspects of accidents as well as the tragic consequences. The case study is an excellent problem solving technique. Normally case studies are presented to a group that has the goal of evaluating the mistakes made in the situation and providing real world solutions. The technique is particularly effective when the group is allowed to come to the conclusion that they can benefit from the mistakes of other construction contractors and thus prevent accidents. Real mishaps are effective case studies and should be used as often as possible to add credibility to the technique, but one must be aware of the sensitivities involved in tragic accidents.

87) Answer C:

The National Institute for Occupational Safety and Health (NIOSH) document "Criteria for a Recommended Standard ... Working in Confined Spaces" provides several recommendations for safely working in confined spaces. Their major recommendations include:

RECOGNITION: Training in what constitutes a confined space and what hazards may be present is essential to the establishment of a good accident prevention system.
TESTING, EVALUATION, AND MONITORING: All confined spaces should be tested by a qualified person before entry. Tests should be made for oxygen, flammability and toxic substances. Evaluation should consider methods of isolation, ventilation, PPE, communication, lockout etc. Monitoring should be continuously employed to determine if the atmosphere has changed while the work is being performed or during breaks in the work routine.
RESCUE: Rescue procedures and training must be well thought out, developed and implemented prior to entry. The rescue procedures should be practiced frequently enough to provide a level of proficiency that eliminates life-threatening rescue attempts and ensure a calm response to any emergency. Advance first-aid training is strongly recommended for all participants in the rescue phase of the operation. Remember that the attendant can not become a rescuer until they have been relieved from their attendant duties. There must be an attendant on duty. The following

example from the NIOSH research file demonstrates the need for an organized confined space entry control program.

Four Fatalities, 40 Hospitalized

A 20 year old construction worker died while attempting to refuel a gasoline engine powered pump used to remove waste water from a 66 inch diameter sewer line that was under construction. The pump was approximately 3,000 feet from where the worker had entered the line. The worker was overcome by carbon monoxide. Two co-workers, who had also entered from another point along the sewer line were also overcome, however one was able to escape. A 28-year-old state inspector entered from another point along the sewer line and died in a rescue attempt. The inspector's apprentice, 21 years of age, was also overcome and died attempting to rescue the inspector. All fatalities were due to carbon monoxide intoxication. In addition to the fatalities, 41 additional rescue, medical and other construction personnel were transported to hospital facilities and treated for carbon monoxide poisoning that occurred while trying to rescue the workers and inspectors. In this example there were serious mistakes made in every phase of operations. In the RECOGNITION phase it is obvious that no one on this job site considered the sewer line a dangerous confined space or was aware of the effects of carbon monoxide. Certainly the TESTING, EVALUATION AND MONITORING, phase was deficient. No one, including the responding rescue team was aware of the concentrations within the sewer line. The RESCUE phase of this mishap produced 40 hospital cases, certainly the rescuers were not prepared for this type of incident. A rapid rescue and proper first aid might have saved all of the fatalities in this tragic incident.

88) Answer A:

OSHA 1926.454 states that the employer shall have each employee who performs work while on a scaffold trained by a person qualified in the subject matter to recognize the hazards associated with the type of scaffold being used and to understand the procedures to control or minimize those hazards. The training shall include the following areas, as applicable:

- The nature of any electrical hazards, fall hazards and falling object hazards in the work area;
- The correct procedures for dealing with electrical hazards and for

erecting, maintaining, and disassembling the fall protection systems and falling object protection systems being used;

- The proper use of the scaffold, and the proper handling of materials on the scaffold;
- The maximum intended load and the load-carrying capacities of the scaffolds used; and
- Any other pertinent requirements of this subpart.

89) Answer B:

According to The Psychology of Safety, while all four answers have an impact on behavior, consequences, in general, have the most impact. Discipline and feedback can be considered types of consequences, but there are others to be considered including positive reinforcement and reward.

90) Answer D:

The OSHA Hazardous Waste Operations and Emergency Response standard, 1910.120, requires general workers to be provided 40 hours of hands-on instruction off-site, combined with at least 3 days field experience under the supervision of a trained supervisor. Additionally, these workers must complete 8 hours of refresher training each 12 months.

91) Answer C:

The three most often recommended fundamental training courses for construction workers are: First Aid, Fire Extinguisher, and Contingency. Contingency meaning emergency procedures.

92) Answer B:

There are three things that will keep a person from listening: Word barriers – e.g. death, liar, layoff, IRS, etc.; Emotional barriers – e.g. bias, boredom, envy, fatigue, etc.; and distractions. A good example of a distraction is to present safety training at the end of a shift. One of the most important times to ensure that training has been presented is before any **non-routine** work.

93) Answer C:

The OSHA Hazard Communication Standard does not cover some materials that come under regulation by government agencies other than OSHA. Included are cosmetics, alcohol, hazardous waste, pesticides and wood products. However, the exemption does not include wood dust and the OSHA PEL for wood dust must be included in the MSDS for such products. Additionally, any wood additives present in the wood, which represent a health hazard must also be included on the MSDSs or label.

94) Answer D:

The benefits of safety and health training include all the following except?

- improved performance
- fewer incidents/accidents
- reduced costs
- reinforcement of the operational goals of the organization

It is not designed to modify attitudes.

95) Answer B:

The strategies listed are below the standard type of instructional strategies.

1. Lecture
2. Demonstration
3. Guided Discussion
4. Individualized Instruction
5. Role Play
6. Learner Discovery Method

96) Answer D:

The instructor should follow the lesson plan and ensure that the trainees meet the objective of the course. The training must meet the trainee's expectation, without an overkill.

97) Answer B:

Reliability is a measure of how well a test item discriminates the knowledge level of the participants. Evaluations for training purposes are **NOT norm-referenced.** Norm-referencing means that how well a trainee scores depends on how well or how poorly other trainees perform. Evaluations for training purposes **should always be criterion-referenced.** This means performance is measured against a pre-set standard. The test must measure what it is supposed to measure. The evaluation tool should always be developed before training begins.

98) Answer A:

The benefits of the lecture is that you can impart information to a large group in a relative short time, however this leaves little time or opportunity for interaction between the trainee and the instructor.

99) Answer C:

The OSHA Hazard Communication Standard requires employees to be provided with the following information and training:

- The requirements of the Hazard Communication Standard.
- Any operations in the work area where hazardous chemicals are present.
- The location and availability of the written hazard communication program, to include the list of chemicals, and material safety data sheets.
- Training on the methods and observations that may be used to detect the presence of release of a hazardous chemical in the work area.
- The physical and health hazards of the chemicals in the work area.
- The measures employees can take to protect themselves from these hazards, including specific procedures such as work practices, emergency procedures, and personal protective equipment.
- The details of the Hazard Communication Program including an explanation of the labeling system and the material safety data sheet, and how employees find and use the information.

100) Answer D:

The following information was extracted from the Hazard Communication Standard "QUIP" published by OSHA. In response to a request for clarification OSHA stated "The HCS sets performance-oriented employee training requirements at section 1926.59 (h) in order to ensure that employees are provided with information and training about the hazardous chemicals they work with, both at the time of their initial assignment and whenever a new hazard is introduced into their work area. However,..., there is no requirement that "employee training records" be maintained at each jobsite, in fact, there is no requirement in the HCS to maintain any records of employee training."

Self-Assessment Exam Two Questions

1) Arrange the following hazard control steps in the proper sequence: (1) guard the hazard (2) engineer the hazard out if possible (3) educate personnel.

    A) 2,1,3.
    B) 3,1,2.
    C) 1,2,3.
    D) 3,2,1.

2) The procedure used to make a job safe by identifying hazards in each step of the job and developing measures to counteract those hazards is called:

    A) MORT analysis.
    B) Fault Tree.
    C) Job Safety Analysis.
    D) Probabilistic Risk Assessment.

3) The ANSI standard that covers construction Hard Hats is:

    A) ANSI Z87.1
    B) ANSI B16.4
    C) ANSI A12.1
    D) ANSI Z89.1

4) Which of the following **best** describes the evaluation of tasks involving steps, hazards and solutions?

    A) System Safety Analysis (SSA).
    B) Fault Tree Analysis (FTA).
    C) Job Safety Analysis (JSA).
    D) Management Oversight and Risk Tree (MORT).

5) Which of the following **best** meets the definition of "Highly Toxic" as described in the OSHA Hazcom standard?

    A) A chemical that causes visible destruction of, or irreversible alterations in, living tissue by chemical action at the site of contact.

    B) A chemical that has a median lethal dose LD 50 of 50 milligrams or less per kilogram of body weight when administered orally to albino rats weighing between 200 and 300 grams each.

    C) A chemical that causes a substantial proportion of exposed people or animals to develop an allergic reaction in normal tissue after repeated exposure to the chemical.

    D) A chemical that has a median lethal dose LD 50 of more than 50 milligrams per kilogram but not more than 500 milligrams per kilogram of body weight when administered orally to albino rats weighing between 200 and 300 grams each..

6) All of the statements shown here are correct about the OSHA Hazard Communication Standard **except?**

    A) Was mandated by Congress through EPA.
    B) Requires hazard evaluation by importers of chemicals.
    C) Requires chemicals to be labeled.
    D) Allows medical personnel access to trade secrets.

7) Which of the following precautions would be the **least effective** against occupational dermatoses?

    A) Frequent washing of the face and hands with an organic solvent followed by soap and water.

    B) Use of good housekeeping and frequent washing with soap and water.

    C) Good hygiene practices and use of gloves.

    D) Frequent washing with soap and water and the use of barrier cream.

8) Which of the following techniques would be the **preferred** control method for preventing exposure to a hazardous noise exposure?

    A) Control employee work hours to reduce exposure time.
    B) Engineer a less hazardous environment.
    C) Provide protective equipment.
    D) Automate the process to reduce worker interaction.

9) Which of the following concerning dilution ventilation is correct?

    A) Controls a contaminant at its source.
    B) Controls fumes from lead fusing.
    C) Controls low toxicity vapors.
    D) Controls asbestos fibers.

10) Which of the following **best** describes the audiogram?

    A) A ear-cleaning machine.
    B) A hearing booth and noise measuring instrument.
    C) A indicator of hearing acuity.
    D) A tool to detect high hazard noise areas.

11) When respirator qualitative fit testing, required by OSHA, is conducted, which of the following is used to perform taste threshold screening?

    A) Isoamyl Acetate.
    B) Isopentyl Acetate.
    C) Banana Oil.
    D) Sodium Saccharin.

12) Which of the following would **not** be required in an OSHA mandated hearing conservation program?

    A) Workers must be provided with hearing protection.
    B) Workers must be trained and retrained annually.
    C) Given an audiogram within 6 months.
    D) Workers must be given time off to protect hearing.

13) Which of the following is **not** a principle benefit of a Job Safety Analysis (JSA)?
    A) Assist the supervisor in training.
    B) Tool to study jobs for possible improvement.
    C) Instruct new personnel on a specific job.
    D) Replaces workplace procedures.

14) Which of the following is **most correct** concerning the safety afforded by building codes?

    A) Building codes ensure safety of all concerned.
    B) Building codes should be considered paramount.
    C) Codes protect construction workers.
    D) Codes represent the minimum requirements for materials and construction.

15) ANSI Z16.2 is designed to provide a standardized method of recording certain accident facts. Which of the following would **not** be included under the provisions of ANSI Z16.2?

    A) Injury classifications.
    B) Accidents not involving injury.
    C) Accident types.
    D) Unsafe Acts.

16) Which of the following is the name of the report that OSHA requires to be posted annually from 1 February to 30 April?

    A) Log and Summary.
    B) Annual Report.
    C) Supplementary record OSHA Form 301.
    D) Summary of Work-Related Injuries and Illnesses, OSHA Form 300A.

17) During most inspections by OSHA the Compliance Officer will calculate the OSHA Lost Work Day Injury (LWDI) rate to use in determining trends. Which of the following categories are included in the OSHA LWDI rate?
    A) Illnesses.
    B) Fatal accidents.
    C) Cases involving days away from work.
    D) First aid injuries.

18) According to the OSHA Standards, how long must the OSHA Form 300 and OSHA Form 301, if used, be kept by the employer?

    A) 1 year after posting.
    B) 3 years after posting.
    C) 5 years after the end of the year to which they relate.
    D) 3 years after the end of the year to which they relate.

19) Employers must report work-related fatalities within eight hours to the nearest OSHA Area Office. What other mishaps would require reporting?

    A) The injury of three or more employee that require medical treatment within 30 days of a work-related incident.
    B) The in-patient hospitalization of three or more employees because of a work-related incident requires reporting within 24 hours.
    C) Any in-patient hospitalization of one or more employee or an amputation because of a work-related incident requires reporting within 24 hours.
    D) The transport of five or more workers to the hospital or any amputation because of a work-related incident requires reporting within 8 hours.

20) The primary reason safety professionals perform accident investigation is to:

    A) Discipline rule violators.
    B) Provide OSHA and the country with valid information.
    C) Satisfy the insurance carrier.
    D) Determine causal conditions.

21) The use of the term *"Accident Proneness"* follows which of the following basic theories?

    A) Accident proneness is a fact of life, we must deal with it but we don't have to like it.
    B) Accident proneness should be identified or discounted early in the mishap investigation process.
    C) Accident prone individuals account for 10% of the work force and about 30% of all accidental loss.
    D) Accident proneness is a concept that has no validity in accident prevention work.

22) Accident costs are generally divided into two areas. What are these two areas?

  A) Budgeted and Non-Budgeted.
  B) Insured and Uninsured.
  C) Direct and Indirect.
  D) Direct and Uninsured.

23) Accidents usually result from:

  A) Personality factors.
  B) Environmental factors.
  C) Physical limitations.
  D) Combinations of factors.

24) Which of the following is the major cause of office accidents?

  A) Falls.
  B) Lack of personal protective equipment.
  C) Struck by falling objects.
  D) Electrical shocks.

25) Accident investigation is done for many reasons. Often several accident investigators will be at the scene of an accident at the same time. Which of the following is the **most important** task with respect to the CHST's accident investigation responsibilities?

  A) Getting to the scene before anybody else.
  B) Preventing the second accident.
  C) Preserving evidence.
  D) Taking care of, or transporting the injured.

26) In an active mishap prevention program who should investigate a serious or fatal accident?

  A) A senior management official.
  B) The safety engineer.
  C) The supervisor.
  D) The insurance investigator.

27) From least important to most important, which of the following indicates the correct order of actions to be taken by an accident investigator?

    A) 1,2,3,4.
    B) 1,3,2,4.
    C) 1,4,2,3.
    D) 1,2,4,3.

    1. Arrive safely
    2. Care for the injured
    3. Size-up the situation
    4. Protect property

28) Which of the following **best** describes the legal premise of "chain of custody"?

    A) Secure storage.
    B) Documentation of possession.
    C) Ownership.
    D) Personal knowledge.

29) Which of the following is **most correct** concerning a rigged object subject to the sudden movement of a hoisting apparatus during a hoisting operation?

    A) The load should be padded.
    B) The load will not be affected.
    C) Stresses will be increased in the rigging.
    D) Safety factors are based on the increased stresses caused by such operations.

30) Which of the following would **most likely** result in the immediate functioning of an electrical magnetic circuit breaker to interrupt the current?

    A) Undersize wiring.
    B) A line-to-line short.
    C) A 20% overload for any period of time.
    D) Ground fault.

31) Which of the following is the **most effective** method of preventing inadvertent startup of electrical equipment that may cause injury or property damage?

    A) Tagout.
    B) Enclosure.
    C) Lockout.
    D) Warning Signs.

32) Which of the following factors does **not** contribute to the depletion of oxygen levels in confined spaces?

    A) Chemical reaction.
    B) Welding.
    C) Bacterial action.
    D) Ventilation.

33) All of the following statements concerning confined space entry are true **except?**

    A) Generally, entry requires respiratory protection.
    B) Ventilation with oxygen is often required.
    C) Rescue plans should be made in advance.
    D) Normally more than one person is required.

34) The OSHA Hazard Communication Standard has limited coverage in several workplaces. In certain instances development and maintenance of a written Hazard Communication Program is not required. Which of the following workplaces falls under this exemption?

    A) Hazardous Waste Sites and Warehouses.
    B) Laboratories and Warehouses.
    C) Convalescent Homes and Warehouses.
    D) Restaurants and Warehouses.

35) According to the OSHA Hazard Communication Standard a material must be listed as a carcinogen on the Safety Data Sheet (SDS) in all of the cases listed below **except?**

   A) If OSHA considers the agent to be a carcinogen then it must be listed as a carcinogen on the SDS.
   B) If the substance is identified as IARC Group 1 it must be listed on the SDS as a carcinogen.
   C) If the substance is identified on the National Toxicology Program "Annual Report on Carcinogens" it must be listed on the SDS.
   D) If the agent was listed in an "in vitro" study as a carcinogen risk.

36) Under the provisions of the OSHA Hazard Communication standard, all of the following would be considered a "health hazard" **except?**

   A) A material with a PEL from OSHA.
   B) A material that poses a ionizing radiation hazard.
   C) A material with a listing in 29 CFR part 1910, subpart Z.
   D) A material with a TLV from ACGIH.

37) All the following would be considered a "health hazard" under the provisions of the OSHA Hazard Communication standard **except?**

   A) Wood products including wood dust.
   B) Hazardous waste under the provisions of RCRA.
   C) A chemical for which there is only one statistically significant study that shows it may produce acute health affects in workers.
   D) A material with a TLV or PEL.

38) You are reviewing the preliminary plans for the construction of a radio transmitting site located at 9,000 feet elevation. The workers will travel from sea level to the site each day and return after 12-hour shifts. Which of the following would you be **most concerned** with?

   A) Caisson disease.
   B) Dequervain's disease.
   C) Raynaud's phenomenon.
   D) Hypoxia.

39) During a pre-job survey of a sub-contractors safety program you discover a disturbing program element. The sub-contractor has performed many Job Safety Analyses (JSAs) to satisfy the legal requirement for a hazard analysis, but the JSAs are then filed and never used in the field. All of the following are valid uses for a JSA **except?**

    A) To provide training for new workers and refresher training for the old hands.

    B) As a survey document when a job or task is modified by new procedures or equipment.

    C) As a replacement for job instructions or workplace procedures.

    D) As a survey instrument to see if a job has changed since last evaluated and to see if the job is currently being performed correctly.

40) Which of the following **best** describes the current definition of *breathing zone*?

    A) A sphere 2 foot in diameter centered on the head.

    B) A sphere 2.2 foot in diameter centered on the head.

    C) A hemisphere 6-9 inches in radius and forward of the shoulders.

    D) A hemisphere 9-18 inches in radius and centered on the shoulder.

41) During review of some pre-planning documents developed by a sub-contractor you notice that the Threshold Limit Values (TLVs) being used are attributed to the American Society of Safety Engineers? What organization has established the TLVs used in industry today?

    A) MSHA.

    B) ACGIH.

    C) ABIH.

    D) AIHA.

42) A sub-contractor is dismantling a tower crane attached to the side of a multi-story building. The tower crane will be disassembled section by section using a mobile crane. Assuming the analysis will be equipment centered, which system safety analysis technique would be the **least effective** for analysis of this project?

    A) Fault Tree Analysis.
    B) Multilinear Events Sequencing.
    C) Job Safety Analysis.
    D) Failure Modes and Effect Analysis.

43) Many injuries on the construction site are caused by material handling accidents. Several techniques have proven to be effective in preventing accidents of this type. Which of the following would be the **least effective** single element in the prevention of materials handling mishaps?

    A) Training.
    B) Stringent physical requirements.
    C) Job placement.
    D) Job descriptions.

44) While checking a general contractor's procedures for first aid medical attention for workers you find the program elements shown below, which one is **not** valid?

    A) First aid will be provided by trained personnel with certificates from the Red Cross.
    B) First aid kits are approved by the supervising occupational physician.
    C) First aid kits are inspected every two weeks by the site safety representative.
    D) The telephone numbers of physicians, hospitals and ambulance service are posted at every job site.

45) Which of the following is a term used to describe the condition *epicondylitis*?

    A) Trigger finger.
    B) Rotator cuff.
    C) Roofer's wrist.
    D) Carpenter's elbow.

46) All of the following actions are required of a company that receives an OSHA citation **except?**
    A) Pay the fine.
    B) Pay the fine and post the notice of violation.
    C) Correct the violation.
    D) Retrain all employees.

47) Which of the following Code of Federal Regulations (CFR) deals with Protection of the Environment?
    A) 10 CFR.
    B) 20 CFR.
    C) 40 CFR.
    D) 42 CFR.

48) The organization established and operated by the American Chemistry Council to provide emergency response information is the:
    A) Chemical Referral Center.
    B) Chemical Emergency Center for Transportation.
    C) Chemical Center for Accident Response Information.
    D) Chemical Transportation Emergency Center.

49) Which act authorizes regulations on the development, distribution, and marketing of chemical substances?
    A) RCRA.
    B) OSHA.
    C) TSCA.
    D) SARA.

50) Any employer who receives a package of hazardous material which is required to be marked, labeled or placarded in accordance with the U. S. Department of Transportation's Hazardous Materials Regulations shall retain those markings, labels and placards on the package until?
    A) 45 days.
    B) Until the container is empty.
    C) Until the container is empty or 90 days, whichever comes first.
    D) The packaging is sufficiently cleaned of residue and purged of vapors to remove any potential hazards.

51) ANSI Z16.2 is designed to provide a standardized method of recording certain accident facts. Which of the following would **not** be included under the provisions of ANSI Z16.2?

    A) Injury classifications.
    B) Hazardous Condition Classification.
    C) Workers Compensation Rating.
    D) Unsafe Acts.

52) OSHA requires that employers keep an OSHA Form 300, "Log of Work-Related Injuries and Illnesses" at each establishment. How current do these logs have to be?

    A) Updated to within 60 days of finding out about an injury or illness.
    B) Updated to within 30 days of finding out about an injury or illness.
    C) Updated to within 14 days of finding out about an injury or illness.
    D) Updated to within 7 days of finding out about an injury or illness.

53) OSHA requires certain posting requirements for the Summary of Work Related Injuries and Illnesses, OSHA Form 300A. What are the requirements for posting if your company did **not** experience any recordable accidents during the year?

    A) Posting is not required.
    B) Post the summary with zeros on the totals line.
    C) Post a signed blank summary.
    D) Complete a summary and file it in case of inspection, posting is not required.

54) On a construction site, at least one portable fire extinguisher having a rating of not less than 20-B units shall be located not less than ___ feet, nor more than ___ feet, from any flammable liquid storage area located outside.

    A) 25, 75.
    B) 25, 100.
    C) 50, 75.
    D) 50, 100.

55) Which of the following were included in Heinrich's 1930's famous domino theory of accidents?
   A) Safety, Security, Belonging, and Self-esteem.
   B) The three E's.
   C) Social, fault, unsafe act, accident, injury.
   D) Man, machine, money, injury, accident.

56) Which of the following would **not** be considered a "health hazard" under the provisions of the OSHA Hazard Communication standard?
   A) A material with a PEL.
   B) A material with a TLV.
   C) A material with a listing in 29 CFR Part 1910, subpart Z.
   D) A material that poses a biological hazard.

57) Which of the following would **not** be considered a "health hazard" under the provisions of the OSHA Hazard Communication standard?
   A) A chemical for which there is only one statistically significant study that shows it may produce acute health affects in workers.
   B) A material with a TLV or PEL.
   C) Wood products including wood dust.
   D) Hazardous waste under the provisions of RCRA.

58) Safety Data Sheets (SDS) must develop evaluation or risk determinations. The procedures used to determine the hazards of the chemical evaluated must be in writing and made available to employees or their designated representatives. Which of the following **best** describes the definition of *designated representative*?
   A) An attorney selected by the employee.
   B) A certified collective bargaining agent.
   C) Another worker selected verbally by the employee.
   D) A foreman or supervisor duly elected by a show of hands.

59) According to OSHA, at what depth must a trench be provided with means of egress such as a stairway, ladder, ramp, etc.?
   A) Greater than 8 feet.
   B) 5 feet or more.
   C) 4 feet or more.
   D) 16 feet or more.

60) In states that have a Right to Know law, the federal OSHA Hazard Communication Standard:
   A) Is preempted.
   B) Preempts the state law in all cases.
   C) Preempts the state law in occupational settings.
   D) Preempts the state law in settings covered by OSHA.

61) Which of the following is incorrect concerning the OSHA hazard communication standard?
   A) Requires hazard evaluation by importers of chemicals.
   B) Was mandated by congress thru EPA.
   C) Requires chemicals to be labeled.
   D) Allows medical personnel access to trade secrets.

62) An overhead crane is equipped with a hoist line limit switch. The purpose of this device is?
   A) To prevent the crane from lifting a weight beyond the load limit.
   B) To prevent the load from being lifted too fast.
   C) To prevent over travel of the load block.
   D) To prevent the crane magnet from being disconnected during lifting.

63) When supplying breathing air to five or more abrasive blasting respirators, what is the minimum amount of air to be supplied to each unit?
   A) 3 CFM.
   B) 6 CFM.
   C) 9 CFM.
   D) 12 CFM.

64) Which of the following **best** describes a Class "B" level of Personal Protective Equipment (PPE)?
   A) Fully-encapsulated chemical-resistant suit with Self Contained Breathing Apparatus (SCBA) or Supplied Air (SA) with escape provisions.
   B) Chemical-resistant suit with Self Contained Breathing Apparatus (SCBA) or Supplied Air (SA) with escape provisions.
   C) Chemical-resistant suit with Air Purifying Respirator (APR).
   D) No chemical protection and no respiratory protection.

65) In 1985 the National Institute for Occupational Safety and Health (NIOSH) convened an ad hoc committee of experts who reviewed the current literature on lifting, recommended criteria for defining lifting capacity, and in 1991 developed a revised lifting equation. The NIOSH 1991 lifting equation contains all of the following **except?**
    A) A coupling multiplier.
    B) A frequency multiplier.
    C) A distance multiplier.
    D) A speed multiplier.

66) The Superfund Amendment and Reauthorization Act (SARA) was the legislative response to the Bhopal tragedy in which 2,000 people were killed and another 200,000 were injured. One of the provisions of SARA was the establishment of several commissions and groups to ensure public dissemination of information and ensure emergency planning is done. The proper name for the emergency committee established at the local level is the _____?
    A) SARA local level committee.
    B) Local Emergency Planning Committee.
    C) Local Level Emergency Planning Commission.
    D) Local Emergency Response Commission.

67) Which of the following is **not** a valid RCRA characteristic of hazardous waste?
    A) Ignitability.
    B) Corrosivity.
    C) Reactivity.
    D) Radioactivity.

68) All of the following concerning flammable inside storage areas are true **except?** Inside storage locations must be provided with:
    A) A clear aisle at least 22 inches wide.
    B) A raised 4-inch sill.
    C) Self-closing fire doors.
    D) Either gravity or mechanical exhaust system.

69) According to 40 CFR, contingency plans must describe arrangements with all the following **except?**

A) State OSHA.
B) Hospitals.
C) Emergency response teams.
D) Disaster teams.

70) The Emergency Planning and Community Right-to-know Act (1986) mandated the creation of the State Emergency Response Committees (SERCs) and the Local Emergency Planning Committees (LEPCs). The LEPC consists of emergency organizations, political entities and companies that meet stated criteria. What is the **most critical** role for companies that manufacture, process or use chemicals that could pose a danger to the local community?

A) Notify committee of a spill or release.
B) Keep committee notified of inventory.
C) Participate in the emergency planning process.
D) Report to the LEPC when chemical levels are above allowable levels.

71) According to 1910.145, which of the following is incorrect when posting a Danger tag?

A) The signal word shall be readable at a minimum distance of 7 feet or greater.
B) The message shall be presented in text or pictographs or both.
C) The tags shall be affixed as close as possible to the hazard.
D) Employees must be informed as to the meaning of the signs.

72) If a radium bearing powder was spilled in your lab, what would be your first action?

A) Report the incident to OSHA.
B) Clean up as quickly as possible.
C) Notify NRC immediately.
D) Evacuate personnel and reroute traffic.

73) The use of industrial robots has risen tremendously in the recent past. The use of these robots creates some additional hazards for workers. Safeguarding must be incorporated in all aspects of design. One of the primary methods of guarding involves the establishment of protection zones or hazard areas. These areas are often called the robot's operating envelope. The primary zone generally deals with hazards involving the maximum designed reach of the robot. The secondary zone includes the area where items could be propelled by the robot if a malfunction should occur. Which of the following statements is **most correct** concerning mishaps involving industrial robots?
A) Most accidents occur during set-up.
B) Most accidents occur within the primary zone of the robot.
C) The vast majority of accidents involved a malfunctioning robot.
D) Most accidents involved unauthorized personnel in or around the hazard zone.

74) Which of the following duties does **not** fall under the provisions of the Toxic Substances Control Act (TOSCA or TSCA)?
A) Required pre-testing of chemicals.
B) Limit import of dangerous chemicals.
C) Limit export.
D) Ban classes of risky chemicals.

75) When preparing for an emergency, the most common plans include all of the following **except?**
A) Action guides/checklist.
B) Response plans.
C) Emergency management plans.
D) Bilateral agreements.

76) When completing a Risk Management Plan (RMP) to comply with CFR 40 (the Clean Air Act of 1970), you must plan for a minimum of ____ scenario(s)?
A) 1.
B) 2.
C) 3..
D) 4

77) When making an environmental audit, it is best to follow a defined set of procedures, sometimes called a protocol. The protocol has three basic areas. Which of the following is **not** considered part of an environmental protocol?
   A) Pre-visit Activities.
   B) Visit Activities.
   C) Determination of liability.
   D) Post-visit Activities.

78) When considering environmental problems, which of the following will have the **least** concern with controlling releases or spills?
   A) The local population.
   B) Company shareholders.
   C) Local suppliers.
   D) Local governmental officials.

79) Under the provisions of the Resource Conservation and Recovery Act (RCRA), generators of hazardous waste have the responsibility to prepare a Uniform Hazardous Waste Manifest which is a transport and control device that stays with the hazardous waste at all times. RCRA also requires generators to maintain copies of the manifest for a period of?
   A) Five years.
   B) Only until delivered and signed for at a TSD.
   C) Three years.
   D) Thirty years.

80) Many small businesses produce hazardous waste that is regulated by the Resource Conservation and Recovery Act (RCRA). If regulated, EPA will control this hazardous waste from the moment it is generated until its ultimate disposal. Which of the following businesses would be considered a small quantity generator by the EPA? You produce more than _____ and less than _____ pounds of hazardous waste in a calendar month.

   A) 200 and 2,000.
   B) 220 and 2,200.
   C) 400 and 4,000.
   D) 440 and 4,400.

81) Section 313 of EPCRA, titled Toxic Chemical Release Reporting (Form R) requires an annual report of all chemicals released to the environment. The report includes all of the following **except?**
   A) The threshold level is 5000 pounds.
   B) All chemicals released as gases, liquids or solids.
   C) The name and CAS number of each chemical.
   D) Location to include the longitude and latitude of the facility.

82) Which of the following **best** describes the main objective of the Toxic Substance Control Act (TSCA)?
   A) Control the distribution of chemicals in the US.
   B) Ensure the quality of our drinking water in the US.
   C) Regulate the production of toxic waste.
   D) Regulate the development and distribution of toxic substances.

83) Under the provisions of the Resource Conservation and Recovery Act (RCRA), containers that have previously held an acutely hazardous waste are considered empty when?
   A) Wastes have been poured out and container turned upside down to drain for 30 minutes or longer.
   B) The container has been triple rinsed with a solvent.
   C) There is no more than 3 inches of residue on the bottom of the container.
   D) The container has been drained and depuddled with sanitary rags.

84) For a single radioactive decay process, the time required for the activity to decrease to half its value by that process is called?
   A) 50% reduction factor.
   B) Radioactive half-life.
   C) Biological half-life.
   D) Radioactive 50% reduction.

85) In accordance with the Toxic Substance Control Act of 1976 (TSCA), which of the following statements is incorrect?

    A) Companies are required to test new chemicals for their acute dermal, inhalation and oral toxic effects.

    B) Companies are required to notify the EPA 120 days before manufacturing a new chemical.

    C) The EPA is authorized to regulate or ban chemical that they deem unsafe.

    D) New chemicals must be tested to determine their effects on the health of individuals and on the environment.

86) According to the OSHA standards, which of the following statements is **most correct** concerning the use of power-operated tools in a construction environment?

    A) Powder-actuated tools must be tested for defects in accordance with manufacturer's recommendations weekly, the test must be recorded and available for inspection.

    B) Airless spray guns above 100 psi must be equipped with a manual safety for operator safety.

    C) Compressed air must be reduced to 30 psi for concrete form cleaning.

    D) Compressed air hoses with a one-half inch inside diameter or greater must have a safety device at the source of supply air to reduce pressure in the event of hose failure.

87) All of the following are recognized classes of protective footwear **except?**

    A) Conductive shoes/boots.

    B) Electrical Hazard Shoes/boots.

    C) Safety-Toe Safety Shoes Class "75".

    D) Non-ionizing, worker Safety Shoe Class "EX" radiation.

88) Which of the following statements is **most correct** concerning the correct shade filter lens during welding & cutting operations?

    A) Generally it is best to pick a #2 lens (dark) and work up, this allows compensation for individual differences.

    B) Heavy gas cutting would require a number 6 to 8 shade lens.

    C) Heavy gas cutting would require a number 14 to 16 shade lens.

    D) As a rule of thumb, it is generally best to start with a lens that gives a clear view of the weld zone and then move up.

89) Which of the following firefighting agents has proven to be the **most effective** in combating Class B fires?

    A) Foam, CO2, Dry Powder.

    B) AFFF, Halon, Dry Chemical.

    C) Halon, Water, Dry Chemical.

    D) Foam, CO2, Dry Chemical.

90) A worker wearing a belt with a six-foot lanyard attached at waist-height could be subject to a maximum of _____ feet free fall?

    A) 6 feet.

    B) 8 feet.

    C) 3 feet.

    D) 9 feet.

91) Complete the following statement. A bench grinder should have the tool rest adjusted to within _____ inch of the wheel, and the tongue guard should be adjusted to within _____ inch of the wheel.

    A) 1/2 inch - 1/2 inch.

    B) 1/4 inch - 1/8 inch.

    C) 1/8 inch - 1/4 inch.

    D) 1/16 inch - 1/4 inch.

92) A standard combustible gas indicator reads in _____ ?

    A) Percentage of LEL.

    B) Tenths of LEL.

    C) Percentage of LFL.

    D) Directly in tenths or hundredths.

93) Which of the following is the **most correct** concerning the OSHA standards for loading of explosives or blasting agents?

    A) The explosive cartridge should fit tightly into vertical drill holes to prevent slippage.

    B) Tamping of explosive charges and primers shall be done with wood or plastic tamping pole without exposed metal or spark producing parts.

    C) Drilling is not permitted within 100 feet of remaining butts of old hoses if there is any suspicion of unexploded charges.

    D) Pickup trucks will not be operated within 50 feet of loaded holes.

94) At least ___ designated person(s) shall be on duty above ground whenever any employee is working underground and shall be responsible for securing immediate aid and keeping an accurate count of employees underground in case of emergency.

    A) None.

    B) One.

    C) Two.

    D) Depends on the size of the underground operation.

95) Which of the following provides the **best** protection when dealing with hoisting and rigging equipment?

    A) Chains, slings and ropes should be inspected before each job.

    B) Hoisting and lifting equipment should be inspected daily.

    C) A thorough inspection of all chains in use shall be made every 18 months.

    D) The use of wire rope that has been bird-caged is permitted for lifting if provided with Crosby clamps every six inches.

96) Which of the following is **not** a required element in the OSHA mandated respirator program?

    A) Training in the use of respirators.

    B) All rescue respirators must be cleaned immediately after use.

    C) Respirators must be inspected at regular intervals.

    D) Respirators must not be used by more than one employee.

97) You are the safety engineer at a large construction site where an excavation is made in Type A soil using a simple slope for protection. The excavation will be open less than 24 hours and is 10 feet in depth. Which of the following **best** describes the requirements of OSHA concerning the horizontal to vertical ratio of the slope?

A) Maximum allowable slope is ½:1.
B) Maximum allowable slope is ¾:1.
C) Maximum allowable slope is 1½:1.
D) Maximum allowable slope is 3:1.

98) Which of the following is an instrument used to measure the air velocity in a ventilation system?

A) Wind rose.
B) Viscometer.
C) Westphal balance.
D) Velometer.

99) An excavation is made in Type C soil using a simple slope for protection. The excavation will be open for greater than 36 hours and is 14 feet in depth. Which of the following **best** describes the requirements of OSHA concerning the horizontal to vertical ratio of the slope?

A) Maximum allowable slope is ½:1.
B) Maximum allowable slope is ¾:1.
C) Maximum allowable slope is 1½:1.
D) Maximum allowable slope is 3:1.

100) Which of the following methods would be used for determining the uptake of lead in the body of a worker?
A) Expired breath analysis for CO.
B) Blood lead level (PhB) and zinc protoporphyrin (ZPP).
C) Urine for Hippuric Acid.
D) Blood test for cholinesterase activity in red cells.

Self-Assessment Exam Two Answers

1) We selected answer A because:

Engineering is always the first, and most successful method of dealing with a problem. Second choice would be to guard the hazard, and last to educate the human element.

2) We selected answer C because:

Means of egress from trench excavations such as a stairway, ladder, ramp or other safe means of egress are required in trench excavations that are 4 feet or more in depth and located so as to require no more than 25 feet of lateral travel for workers. OSHA 1926.651.

3) We selected answer D because:

ANSI Z 87.1 deals with Occupational and Educational Eye and Face Protection. *ANSI Z 16.4* concern Uniform Recordkeeping for Occupational Injuries and Illnesses. *ANSI A 12.1* is the standard for Floor and Wall Openings, Railings, and Toeboards. **ANSI Z 89.1** is the authority on Protective Headgear for Industrial Workers.

4) We selected answer C because:

Job Safety Analysis is a systematic analysis of job elements. It results in an in-depth evaluation by workers and first line supervisors of the individual steps and hazards. JSAs also offer protective measures or solutions to identified hazards. Option "A" (System Safety Analysis) is a broad term covering all of the various system safety tools used in the analysis of system risk. Option "B", Fault Tree Analysis is the process of using deductive logic to determine the combination of events that caused a hazardous event to occur. It normally is accompanied by a companion report that evaluates the overall likelihood of failure and provides solutions to the findings discovered in FTA. Option "D" MORT, Management Oversight and Risk Tree is a formal decision tree used in the evaluation of safety programs or as an accident investigation tool. The tool is exhaustive, offering about 1500 events to be evaluated. For this reason it is often considered overkill for all but the largest evaluations or mishaps. However, the system logic is sound and recently several practitioners have produced mini-mort charts that have proven to be useful tools for smaller applications.

5) We selected answer B because:

OSHA at 1910.1200 Appendix A provides definitions for various terms. Selection "A" is the definition of a "Corrosive Chemical". Selection "C" defines a "Sensitizer" and selection "D" provided the definition for "Toxic".

6) We selected answer A because:

The Hazard Communication Standard sometimes referred as the Right-to-know law, is a Standard (1926.59) issued by *OSHA*. It establishes controls over chemicals used in the workplace which include:

- Hazard evaluation by the chemical manufactures and importers
- Provisions for allowing medical personnel access to trade secrets in the event of an exposure or non-emergency
- Establishment of a HAZCOM program to label containers, provide material safety data sheets, and train employees of the hazards of chemicals they work with or may come into contact

The EPA is not involved in regulations dealing with the Hazard Communication Standard.

OSHA normally requires the chemical manufacturer or importer to evaluate chemicals and determine if they present a health hazard. However, it is permissible for the employer to perform the evaluation.

7) We selected answer A because:

Washing with solvent is not a recommended practice and has a high probability of creating dermatoses.

8) We selected answer B because:

Of the various methods available to the Construction Health and Safety Technician, *Engineering* controls are by far the preferred method. This would include initial design or by using the techniques of substitution, ventilation or isolation. *Administrative* controls that provide control of the workers exposure are next in prevention value. *Personal Protective Equipment* is the last resort to provide worker protection.

9) We selected answer C because:

Dilution ventilation lowers the concentration of a contaminant by adding air to the general work area. Since the air is added to the general work area it will not effectively control exposure to a toxic or highly toxic substance used in a specific location.

10) We selected answer C because:

An audiogram is a record of hearing loss or hearing level measured at several different frequencies, normally from 500 to 6000 hertz. Hearing levels are generally presented graphically as a function of frequency. The audiogram measures the acuity or sharpness of hearing ability.

11) We selected answer D because:

Taste threshold screening is conducted using a solution of 0.83 grams of *sodium saccharin* in water. Safety and Health Practitioners preparing for the CHST examination should become familiar with all of the Qualitative Fit Test Protocols required by OSHA.

12) We selected answer D because:

The OSHA requirements include provisions for insuring that the employees are provided hearing protection, given a baseline hearing test (audiogram) in most cases the audiogram is required within 6 months. However requirements for removal from the industrial environment to protect hearing is required only after a hearing threshold shift is detected.

13) We selected answer D because:

The principle benefits of a Job Safety Analysis (JSA) are:

- Allowing the supervisor to perform training for safe, efficient operations
- Allowing the supervisor or other person developing the JSA to meet and work with employees
- Instruction of new employees on specific jobs
- Instruction of current employees on the specifics of jobs performed

irregularly
- As an accident investigation tool should a mishap occur
- Studying jobs to determine if improvement is possible

14)   We selected answer D because:

Building codes are designed to protect the future occupants of the building and offer little protection for the actual construction workers. Because codes attempt to predict the future use of the building they are considered the *absolute minimum protection* requirements.

15)   We selected answer B because:

ANSI Z16.2 does not include any provisions for recording details about mishaps that did not produce an injury. That is, an event that did not result in physical harm to a person.

16)   We selected answer D because:

Most employers covered under OSHA are required to maintain records of injuries and illnesses. The Summary of Work-Related Injuries and Illnesses shall be posted from 1 February to 30 April each year.

17)   We selected answer C because:

The LWDI (lost-workday-injury-rate) considers only injuries, illnesses are not included. Fatalities are not included nor are first aid injuries that do not require medical treatment of a recurring nature. The LWDI has served as a benchmark for OSHA in the past. Should a company receive a programmed inspection, an initial review of records will include an evaluation of the LWDI. If the rate is below the average LWDI for that SIC (Standard Industry Classification) then the company might not have to submit to a full inspection. However, if the LWDI is above the average a full inspection is almost certain. Although cases of illnesses are not used in the calculation of the LWDI, the OSHA CSHO conducting a safety inspection will probably make note of any significant recorded illnesses and submit a health referral if appropriate.

18)   We selected answer C because:

OSHA Standard 1904 requires that the OSHA Form 301 and 300 be kept in each establishment for 5 years following the end of the year to which they relate.

19) We selected answer C because:

As of January 1, 2015, all employers must report:

- All work-related fatalities within 8 hours.
- All work-related inpatient hospitalizations within 24 hours,
- All amputations and all losses of an eye within 24 hours.

The employer of any employees so affected shall orally report the fatality/in-patient hospitalization by telephone or in person to the Area Office of the Occupational Safety and Health Administration (OSHA), U.S. Department of Labor, that is nearest to the site of the incident, or by using the OSHA toll-free central telephone number.

This requirement applies to each such fatality or hospitalization of one or more employees, which occurs within thirty days of an incident.

Exception: If the employer does not learn of a reportable incident at the time it occurs and the incident would otherwise be reportable, as defined above, the employer shall make the report within 8 hours of the time the incident is reported to any agent or employee of the employer.

Each report required by this section shall relate the following information:

- Establishment name
- location of incident
- time of the incident
- number of fatalities or hospitalized employees
- names of injured employees
- contact person
- phone number
- description of incident

20) We selected answer D because:

Accidents or mishaps are investigated by safety and health professionals to determine the root cause factors and to prevent future occurrences of the same type by implementing appropriate corrective actions. This goal must be kept in mind throughout the investigation process. Many times other investigations are being conducted for other reasons, for example, security, personnel or possibly even the legal staff may be interested in facts surrounding any unusual event. These investigations usually are searching for discipline, reimbursement, protection from liability/litigation or the assessment of blame. It is not uncommon for the safety professional to be drawn into these investigations because of their investigative skills and in-depth knowledge of the job site. However, it is imperative that accident prevention investigations be separated from discipline investigations if one is to find the true cause factors. Firing the person who had the accident, rarely will prevent the next one.

21) We selected answer D because:

Current thinking within the safety community follows the belief that accident proneness is not a proven scientific fact but rather unfounded hypotheses designed to explain the behavior of humans. The theory is rejected in virtually all safety work.

22) We selected answer C because:

Accident costs have for many years been divided into direct and indirect costs. Direct costs are those costs directly and often immediately associated with the accident such as: transportation of the injured, medical services, days lost from work etc. Indirect costs would include: lost production, replacement of the injured worker, costs of training a replacement etc. **The indirect costs associated with accidents rarely consider the effects of a mishap on family members.**

23) We selected answer D because:

Accidents are usually multi-causal in nature and cannot be attributed entirely to any single factor.

24) We selected answer A because:

Falls are by far the most common cause of office mishaps.

25) We selected answer B because:

There is no doubt that an investigator's first tasking is to get to the scene safely. Everyone is in a hurry to get to the scene of the accident, but you cannot render assistance or perform an adequate investigation if you do not arrive safely. The job of a health and safety professional cannot start until the scene is secured, meaning that the injured are taken care of and the scene itself is made safe. If you arrive earlier than this you run the risk of becoming part of the emergency services effort which tends to make you part of the response rather than part of the investigative team. There are exceptions, such as in the care of the safety engineer who is part of the rescue or re-entry team, but in most cases the advice is solid.

26) We selected answer A because:

Senior management should investigate:

- Fatal accidents
- Accidents with large losses or the potential for large losses
- Mishaps that result or could result in adverse public reaction

Lower levels of supervision and the safety director/engineer should also be involved in these investigations. The safety engineer should act as the company resident expert in mishap investigation procedures and techniques offering advice and possibly training to other members of the investigation team. Most progressive companies also provide a standardized accident investigation "system" to be used on all important or large mishap investigations. The systems are varied and take many forms. They may be as simple as a checklist of items to be examined with a cause and effect report format or an extensive system that details the entire investigative effort from membership to analysis to formal reporting with corporate presentations.

27) We selected answer B because:

It is generally accepted within the health and safety community that the order of sequence for accident investigation should be:

- Arrive safely

  You cannot do anyone any good if you are involved in an accident yourself racing to the scene of a tragedy. Once on the scene, **isolate it and control the access** to prevent further mishaps.

- Size up

The professional fire service uses the term "size-up" to indicate the time spent observing and analyzing the event. The same tactic should be used by investigators to determine what evidence must be protected, who is involved, who is on the scene, is the site now safe or is another mishap about to occur etc. Experience will allow you to accomplish this task very fast.

- Care for injured

    If necessary the investigator should help injured and protect property. However, the investigators job is to gather facts not provide emergency service. Generally this job is best left to others. It is fine to render aid if you are needed but don't get in the way of the professionals.

- Protect property

    Prevention of the second accident is an important aspect of the accident investigators job. Because of their observation skills and training, safety professionals can often spot unsafe conditions that others involved in the emergency will not see. You must above all else, not allow an accident to escalate into a disaster.

28) We selected answer B because:

Often if evidence is to be used in a court of law the chain of custody must be documented. The chain of custody is simply a documented explanation of where the evidence was obtained and where it has been since that time. The evidence must have been secured from tampering or change. The court must be assured through the chain of custody that the evidence is unchanged or changes can be explained.

29) We selected answer C because:

The inertia of an object in motion that takes place when an increase or decrease in speed causes great increases in stress on the rigging. As a load line starts to move sudden accelerations can cause as much as twice the stress on the rigging as the actual load. This is why most rigging or hoisting instructions contain warnings or cautions about applying lifting forces in a slow and smooth manner.

30) We selected answer B because:

This question seeks a situation that would *most likely* cause immediate functioning of a magnetic circuit breaker. The situation that qualifies is a line-to-line short. Undersize wiring would most likely result in an overload sufficient to operate the circuit breaker but only after a period of time (unless the wiring was grossly undersized). A 20% overload *might* operate the circuit breaker depending on other conditions. A ground fault would not operate the circuit breaker unless the ground fault resulted in a overload.

31) We selected answer C because:

The Control of Hazardous Energy is a fundamental accident prevention control program that affects the control of all potential and kinetic energy (not just electrical). It is addressed in great detail in OSHA at 1910.147. The most effective method of preventing inadvertent startup of equipment is to provide a substantial lock with rigid key control, combined with a tag and education of all personnel involved.

32) We selected answer D because:

The oxygen levels in confined space can decrease for many reasons, some not readily apparent to the person about to make entry. For example, the oxygen levels could decrease due to the nature of operations being conducted i.e.; welding, cutting, brazing etc. Certain chemical reactions (rusting) can cause an oxygen shortage or bacterial action (fermentation) can reduce the oxygen levels. *Ventilation* would not reduce the oxygen level although it would aid in the mixing process.

33) We selected answer B because:

Never use oxygen to ventilate a confined space. An oxygen-enriched atmosphere will cause flammable materials, such as your clothing and hair to burn violently if ignited. All ventilation should be done with clean dry air. The other choices are all true. Respiratory protection is frequently needed for confined space entry. Over 50% of the workers who die in confined spaces are attempting to rescue other workers. Rescuers must be trained in and follow established emergency procedures and use appropriate equipment and techniques. Rescue plans should be made well in advance of any actual entry and a standby person should be assigned to remain on the outside of the confined space and be in constant contact with the workers inside.

34) We selected answer B because:

There are two types of work operations where the coverage of the Hazard Communication Standard is limited. These are laboratories and operations where chemicals are only handled in sealed containers, eg: a warehouse. Employers having these types of work operations need only:

- keep labels on containers as they are received
- maintain material safety data sheets that are received, and give employees access to them
- provide information and training for employees

Employers do not have to have written hazard communication programs and lists of chemicals for these types of operations.

35) We selected answer D because:

OSHA states "Chemical manufacturers, importers and employers evaluating chemicals shall treat the following sources as establishing that a chemical is a carcinogen or potential carcinogen for hazard communication purposes:

- National Toxicology Program (NTP), "Annual Report on Carcinogens" (latest edition)
- International Agency for Research on Cancer (IARC) "Monographs" (latest edition)
- 29 CFR part 1910, subpart Z, Toxic and Hazardous Substances"

Note: The "Registry of Toxic Effects of Chemical Substances" published by the National Institute for Occupational Safety and Health (NIOSH) indicates whether a chemical has been found by NTP or IARC to be a potential carcinogen.

The IARC provides a summary classification of a chemical's carcinogenic risk according to the following table:

Group1	The agent is carcinogenic to humans
Group2A	The agent is probably carcinogenic to humans
Group2B	The agent is possibly carcinogenic to humans
Group3	The agent is not classifiable as to its carcinogenicity to

humans

Group4   The agent is probably not carcinogenic to humans

All IARC listed chemicals in Groups 1 and 2A must include appropriate entries on both the MSDSs and on the label. Group 2B chemicals need be noted only on the MSDSs.

The use of in vitro (short term) testing (such as the Ames assay) has not been specifically addressed in the Hazard Communication Standard. However, it is the consensus within OSHA that the results of an "in vitro" test alone, does not represent significant enough information to establish a health hazard for purposes of the hazard communication standard.

36)   We selected answer B because:

OSHA classifies as a "health hazard" any chemical for which the American Conference of Governmental Industrial Hygienists (ACGIH) has established a Threshold Limit Value (TLV), any chemical for which OSHA has established a Permissible Exposure Limit (PEL), or listed in 29 CFR Part 1910, subpart Z, Toxic and Hazardous Substances. Biological hazards, ionizing and non-ionizing radiation are not included in the definition of health hazards for purposes of the Hazard Communication Standard.

37)   We selected answer B because:

Selection "A" is partially correct, wood products are not included in the Hazard Communication Standard however the wood and wood products exemption was never intended by OSHA to exclude wood dust from coverage. There is significant evidence that indicates wood dust presents a carcinogenic hazard when inhaled by exposed workers. Thus where there are work operations that generate respirable wood dust, it is appropriate to ensure that workers avoid inhalation and are apprised of the possible carcinogenic hazards. Further, any chemical additives present in the wood, which represent a health hazard must also be included on the MSDSs and/or label as appropriate. Selection "B" is the best choice, because OSHA does not regulate any hazardous waste as defined by the Resource Conservation and Recovery Act (RCRA). Selection "C" is true OSHA classifies as a "health hazard" any chemical for which there is statistically significant evidence based on at least one study conducted in accordance with scientific principles, that acute or chronic health effects may occur in exposed employees. Selection "D" is also true, OSHA classifies as a "health hazard" any chemical for which the American Conference of Governmental Industrial Hygienists (ACGIH) has established a Threshold Limit Value (TLV), any chemical for which OSHA has established a Permissible Exposure Limit (PEL), or listed in 29 CFR Part 1910, subpart Z, Toxic and Hazardous Substances.

38) We selected answer D because:

Hypoxia is caused by lack of oxygen and can be experienced by industrial workers in extreme elevations under heavy workloads or in confined spaces with oxygen deficiencies. Selection "A", Caisson disease or decompression sickness, could be experienced in divers or other high pressure environments. One example is underwater tunnels where pressure is maintained to avoid the affects of water leaking into the heading. Selection "B", is a disorder from the narrowing of the tendon sheath for the abductor muscles of the thumb. Dequervain disease is often seen in workers who perform manual tasks requiring firm grips. Selection "C", Raynaud's phenomenon, is sometimes called white finger and results from a combination of cold and vibration.

39) We selected answer C because:

Job Safety Analysis is a systematic analysis of job elements. It results in an in-depth evaluation by workers and first line supervisors of the individual steps and hazards. JSAs also offer protective measures or solutions to identified hazards. The principle benefits of a Job Safety Analysis (JSA) are:

- Allowing the supervisor to perform training is safe, efficient operations
- Allowing the supervisor or other person developing the JSA to meet and work with employees
- Instruction of new employees on specific jobs
- Instruction of current employees on the specifics of jobs performed irregularly
- As an accident investigation tool should a mishap occur
- Studying jobs to determine if improvement is possible

40)   We selected answer C because:

The preferred definition of Breathing Zone is a hemisphere forward of the shoulders with a radius of approximately 6 to 9 inches.

41)   We selected answer B because:

The American Conference of Governmental Industrial Hygienists (ACGIH) establishes the "TLV" values commonly in use today.

The Threshold Limit Values (TLVs) and Biological Exposure Indices (BEIs) are developed as guidelines to assist in the control of health hazards. They are intended for use in the practice of Industrial Hygiene and should be interpreted and applied only by trained personnel.

42)   We selected answer C because:

Of the techniques listed for answers in this question, Job Safety Analysis would be the least effective. JSA tends to be too task oriented to be used successfully in a very complex operation.

43)   We selected answer D because:

According to leading authorities, most materials handling accidents can be prevented by the establishment of several standard program elements. Included among these elements is training on the hazards of improper movement of materials, lifting techniques and proper conditioning. The establishment of physical requirements for strenuous materials handling applications has proven to be a valuable mishap reduction technique. Likewise, proper job placement is important in any area but certainly in the area of materials handling. Job descriptions as a single program element will not produce any appreciable effect on mishaps.

44)   We selected answer C because:

As required by OSHA first aid kits must be checked before being sent out on each job and on the job at least weekly to make sure expended items are replaced. Additionally, the kits must be weatherproof with each item individually sealed and must be readily accessible on the job site.

45) We selected answer D because:

The disorder "epicondylitis" is often called tennis elbow or sometimes carpenter's elbow. The disorder is a result of combined motion causing pronation of the hand and ulnar deviation. For a carpenter this involves swinging heavy hammers and in tennis swinging the racket. The affliction causes considerable pain in the hand, forearm and elbow. The term *rotator cuff* is associated with the tearing of a ligament in the shoulder. *Roofer's wrist* is a common name for carpal tunnel syndrome which is a disorder caused by compression of the median nerve. *Trigger finger* is an affliction caused by repeated use of the finger pulling levers or triggers, e.g.: paint spray operators.

46) We selected answer D because:

Training of employees may not be required by every citation issued by OSHA.

47) We selected answer C because:

The CFRs are organized under 50 titles each dealing with broad subject areas of federal regulation. Protection of the environment is covered in 40 CFR.

48) We selected answer D because:

CHEMTREC the acronym for Chemical Transportation Emergency Center is a 24-hour telephone center operated by the American Chemistry Council that provides assistance in response to HAZMAT incidents in transportation.

49) We selected answer C because:

The Toxic Substances Control Act (TSCA), as the name implies, deals with the development and distribution of new chemicals introduced into the workplace within the United States.

50) We selected answer D because:

1910.1201 or 1926.61 Any employer who receives a package of hazardous material which is required to be marked, labeled or placarded in accordance with the U. S. Department of Transportation's Hazardous Materials Regulations (49 CFR Parts 171 through 180) shall retain those markings, labels and placards on the package until the packaging is sufficiently cleaned of residue and purged of vapors to remove any potential hazards. Any employer who receives a freight container, rail freight car, motor vehicle, or transport vehicle that is required to be marked or placarded in accordance with the Hazardous Materials Regulations shall retain those markings and placards on the freight container, rail freight car, motor vehicle or transport vehicle until the hazardous materials which require the marking or placarding are sufficiently removed to prevent any potential hazards. Markings, placards and labels shall be maintained in a manner that ensures that they are readily visible. For non-bulk packages which will not be reshipped, the provisions of this section are met if a label or other acceptable marking is affixed in accordance with the Hazard Communication Standard (29 CFR 1910.1200).

51)   We selected answer C because:

ANSI Z16.2 does not include any provisions for recording workers compensation information. The classifications that are included are:

- Nature of Injury
- Part of Body Affected
- Source of Injury
- Accident Type
- Hazardous Condition
- Agency of Accident
- Agency of Accident Part
- Unsafe Act

52)   We selected answer D because:

OSHA Standard 1904 requires employers to maintain in each establishment a log and summary of all recordable occupational injuries and illnesses for that establishment and update the log not later than 7 working days after receiving information that a injury or illness has occurred. Substitutes for the OSHA Form 300, "Log of Work-Related Injuries and Illnesses" are acceptable and some exceptions for maintenance of the data is provided in the standard for multi-location worksites.

53) We selected answer B because:

The Summary of Work-Related Injuries and Illnesses, OSHA Form 300A is to be posted from 1 February to 30 April each year. If no injuries or illnesses occurred in the year, zeros must be entered on the totals line, and the form must be posted. All forms must be certified by a company official.

54) We selected answer A because:

1926.152(d) "Fire control for flammable or combustible liquid storage." At least one portable fire extinguisher, having a rating of not less than 20-B units, shall be located outside of, but not more than 10 feet from, the door opening into any room used for storage of more than 60 gallons of flammable or combustible liquids.
At least one portable fire extinguisher having a rating of not less than 20-B units shall be located not less than 25 feet, nor more than 75 feet, from any flammable liquid storage area located outside.

55) We selected answer C because:

The correct answer is social, fault, unsafe act, accident, injury.

56) We selected answer D because:

OSHA classifies as a "health hazard" any chemical for which the American Conference of Governmental Industrial Hygienists (ACGIH) has established a Threshold Limit Value (TLV), any chemical for which OSHA has established a Permissible Exposure Limit (PEL), or listed in 29 CFR part 1910, subpart Z, Toxic and Hazardous Substances. Biological hazards, ionizing and non-ionizing radiation are not included in the definition of health hazards for purposes of the Hazard Communication Standard.

57) We selected answer D because:

Selection "A" is true. OSHA classifies as a "health hazard" any chemical for which there is statistically significant evidence based on at least one study conducted in accordance with scientific principles, that acute or chronic health effects may occur in exposed employees. Selection "B" is also true, OSHA classifies as a "health hazard" any chemical for which the American Conference of Governmental Industrial Hygienists (ACGIH) has established a Threshold Limit Value (TLV), any chemical for which OSHA has established a Permissible Exposure Limit (PEL), or listed in 29 CFR part 1910, subpart Z, Toxic and Hazardous Substances. Selection "C" is almost correct, wood products are not included in the Hazard Communication Standard however the wood and wood products exemption was never intended by OSHA to exclude wood dust from coverage. There is significant evidence that indicates wood dust presents a carcinogenic hazard when inhaled by exposed workers. Thus where there are work operations that generate respirable wood dust, it is appropriate to ensure that workers avoid inhalation and are apprised of the possible carcinogenic hazards. Further, any chemical additives present in the wood, which represent a health hazard must also be included on the MSDSs and/or label as appropriate. Biological hazards, ionizing and non-ionizing radiation are not included in the definition of health hazards for purposes of the Hazard Communication Standard. Selection "D" is the best choice, because OSHA does not regulate any hazardous waste as defined by the Resource Conservation and Recovery Act (RCRA).

58) We selected answer B because:

OSHA defines a designated representative as an individual or organization to whom an employee gives written authorization to exercise employee's rights under the Hazard Communication standard. A recognized or certified collective bargaining agent shall be treated automatically as a designated representative without regard to written employee authorization.

59) We selected answer A because:

There are two types of work operations where the coverage of the Hazard Communication Standard is limited. These are laboratories and operations where chemicals are only handled in sealed containers ie; a warehouse. Employers having these types of work operations need only keep labels on containers as they are received; maintain material safety data sheets that are received, and give employees access to them; and provide information and training for employees. Employers do not have to have written hazard communication programs and lists of chemical for these types of operations.

60) We selected answer D because:

The Federal Hazard Communication Standard preempts the state law where the two laws conflict.

61) We selected answer B because:

The Hazard Communication Standard, sometimes referred as the Right-to-Know Law, is a Standard (1926.59) issued by OSHA. It establishes controls over chemicals used in the workplace which include:

- Hazard evaluation by the chemical manufacturers and importers
- Provisions for allowing medical personnel access to trade secrets in the event of an exposure or non-emergency
- Establishment of a HAZCOM program to label containers, provide material safety data sheets, and train employees of the hazards of chemicals they work with or may come into contact

The EPA is not involved in regulations dealing with the Hazard Communication Standard. OSHA normally requires the chemical manufacturer or importer to evaluate chemicals and determine if they present a health hazard. However, it is permissible for the employer to perform the evaluation.

62) We selected answer C because:

Overhead cranes can be equipped with several types of limit switches. However, the only valid choice in this selection is to prevent the over travel of the load block. This prevents the load block from being drawn into the sheave or drums and is often referred to as an anti-two block device. In the illustration shown here a switch is attached to the crane boom. The switch is held in the closed position by a weight that slides down the hoisting line. When the load block comes too close to the point sheave the weight is lifted and allows the spring- loaded switch to open and disconnect power to the hoist motor.

63) We selected answer B because:

Respirable air under suitable pressure should be delivered to each respirator at a volume of at least 6 CFM.

64) We selected answer B because:

Modified Chart of EPA/OSHA Levels of Protection			
Levels	Skin	Respiratory	When
A	Fully-encapsulating, chemical-resistant suit, inner gloves, chemical-resistant safety boots.	Pressure-demand, full-facepiece SCBA or pressure-demand supplied-air respirator with escape SCBA.	Highest level of protection indicated by high concentration of atmospheric vapors, gases or particulates or splash hazard exists.
B	Chemical-resistant clothing (overalls and long-sleeved jacket; hooded, one or two piece chemical splash suit; disposable chemical-resistant one-piece suit), inner and outer gloves, chemical resistant safety boots and hard hat.	Pressure-demand, full-facepiece SCBA or pressure-demand supplied-air respirator with escape SCBA.	High level of respiratory protection required, but less skin protection. IDLH, less than 19.5% oxygen.
C	Chemical-resistant clothing (overalls and long-sleeved jacket; hooded, one or two piece chemical splash suit; disposable chemical-resistant one-piece suit), inner and outer gloves, chemical resistant safety boots and hard hat.	Full-facepiece, air-purifying, canister-equipped respirator.	The contaminants, splashes, or direct contact will not affect exposed flesh. Canister will remove contaminant.
D	Overalls, Safety Boots, safety glasses or chemical splash goggles, hardhat.	No respiratory protection and minimal skin protection.	The atmosphere contains no known hazard. Splashes, immersion or inhalation improbable

65) We selected answer D because:

The 1991 NIOSH lifting equation is expressed as:

$$RWL = LC \times HM \times VM \times DM \times AM \times FM \times CM$$

LC = load constant
HM = horizontal multiplier
VM = vertical multiplier
DM = distance multiplier
AM = asymmetric multiplier
FM = frequency multiplier
CM = coupling multiplier

H= Horizontal distance of hand from midpoint between the ankles.
V= Vertical distance from the hands to the floor.
D=Vertical travel distance between the origin and the destination of the lift
A=Angle of asymmetry - angular displacement of the load from the sagittal plane.
F=Average frequency rate of lifting measured in lifts/min.
C=Type of grip attained on object to be lifted.

66) We selected answer B because:

SARA requires each state governor appoint a state emergency response commission (SERC). This commission provided oversight of the local committees, which they appoint. The SERC appoints and supervises *Local Emergency Planning Committees* which are made up of:

- Fire, civil defense, police and public health and safety officials
- Elected state and local officials
- Environmental, emergency preparedness, safety, hospital and transportation officials
- Community groups and representatives from companies and plants affected by the SARA requirements

The LEPC must prepare an emergency plan that contains, at a minimum, the following.

a. Identification of facilities within the emergency planning district, including institutions that contribute risk by their location
b. Methods and procedures for responding to a release
c. Designation of community and facility emergency coordinators
d. Procedures for notification of public and response team
e. How to determine if a release has occurred and affected area
f. Available emergency equipment and personnel
g. Evacuation plans
h. Training programs

      i.   Emergency planning exercises

This plan must be agreed to by the emergency services providers. When communities, fire departments or industrial plants are organized to assist other members in the event of an emergency or disaster, the relationship is known as a "mutual aid plan".

67)   We selected answer D because:

The Resource Conservation and Recovery Act (RCRA) requires that all waste be classified prior to handling. The waste is considered hazardous if it meets certain conditions or exhibits certain characteristics including tests for:

- Ignitability
- Corrosivity
- Reactivity
- Toxicity

68)   We selected answer A because:

Storage using inside storage rooms must normally comply with NFPA 30 which requires that every inside storage room be equipped with one clear aisle at least three feet wide, not 22 inches as specified in answer selection "A". The standard also requires a raised 4 inch sill to prevent run off of any spilled material, self-closing fire doors and some type of exhaust system.

69)   We selected answer A because:

Reference 40 CFR 256.52. When arrangements have been coordinated with the required agencies, the local fire department will normally be designated the incident commander, because of their greater experience, more equipment and training levels than the facility staff.

70)   We selected answer C because:

The most important step is to ensure that the Emergency Plan has all the data from the local companies to ensure that they are accounted for during the planning process.

71)   We selected answer A because:

The required difference for readability is "5" feet. The use of both written text and pictographs will ensure understanding in a culturally diverse work force. Additionally, signs should be in positive terms, should be in concise easy to read terms, warn against potential hazards and signs for the same type of situation should not vary in design at the same location.

72) We selected answer D because:

If radioactive materials that emit alpha particles such as radium, are spilled, if they leak out of their container, or if they are involved in a fire, it is easy to spread them over a large area and thus create major problems. The first step when you have an accident is to protect personnel and property from further damage.

73) We selected answer B because:

Several studies of accidents involving robots have been conducted both in the United States and in Japan. The most often cited accident involved programming, teaching and maintenance. All of these functions are performed within the primary operating envelope of the robot. The greatest risk is during the teach mode when a person must closely observe the movements of the robot to insure close tolerance capability. Alternately, a person might actually guide the robot manipulator through a series of complicated movements while a feedback computer stores the actions. Generally only one person is allowed within the operating envelope during initial teaching sessions. A dead man or pendant control is required during these sessions. There were no instances in any of the studies of injuries to unauthorized personnel.

74) We selected answer C because:

The Toxic Substances Control Act requires the EPA to regulate any substance that "may pose an unreasonable risk of injury to health or the environment". The EPA is also charged with determining what is unreasonable. This charge includes: Under the broad category of regulating the elements of development; manufacturing, distribution and marketing. Additionally, specified chemicals must be tested to determine their effects on the environment.

75) We selected answer D because:

The most common type of plans used in industry today are the-

- action guides/checklist
- response plans
- emergency management plans
- mutual aid plans

Mutual aid plans with neighboring companies and community agencies should include establishing an organizational structure and communication system. Evaluating emergency scenarios requires one to consider not only the types of loss events that can occur, but how the loss events will affect the organization. Loss events can involve frequent, low consequence events and rare, high consequence events. Understanding the risk of each of these loss events is critical for understanding the necessary response to emergency scenarios.

76) We selected answer A because:

40 CFR Sec. 68.25 Worst-case release scenario analysis.

(a) The owner or operator shall analyze and report in the RMP:
(1)For Program 1 processes, one worst-case release scenario for each Program 1 process;
(2) For Program 2 and 3 processes:
One worst-case release scenario that is estimated to create the greatest distance in any direction to an endpoint provided in appendix A of this part resulting from an accidental release of regulated toxic substances from covered processes under worst-case conditions defined in Sec. 68.22;
One worst-case release scenario that is estimated to create the greatest distance in any direction to an endpoint defined in Sec. 68.22(a) resulting from an accidental release of regulated flammable substances from covered processes under worst-case conditions defined in Sec. 68.22; and
Additional worst-case release scenarios for a hazard class if a worst-case release from another covered process at the stationary source potentially affects public receptors different from those potentially affected by the worst-case release scenario developed under paragraphs (a)(2)(i) or (a)(2)(ii) of this section.

77) We selected answer C because:

According to the NSC Environmental Management Accident Prevention Manual, the Environmental Audit Protocol consists of three parts, the pre-visit, where you establish contact, prepare the questionnaire and establish reporting relationships. During the visit phase, conduct the entrance briefing, tour the facility, record, interview, review records, inspect, record findings and have an exit briefing. During the post activity, follow up to resolve outstanding issues and provide audit reports. Determining liability is not part of the audit protocol.

78) We selected answer B because:

Generally, concern is higher among individuals and organizations that may be directly affected by the spill or release. The term NIMBY (not in my backyard) has been applied to the local population that has the most concern.

79) We selected answer C because:

RCRA requires a cradle to grave system of hazardous waste management and one of the items required is the hazardous waste manifest. The hazardous waste manifest must be prepared by the generator, in sufficient copies, so that everyone handling the waste will get a copy. A final copy will be returned to the generator by the TSD who must by force of law retain a copy for three years. If after 45 days, the generator has not heard from the TSD, a notice of exception must be filed with EPA. The notice must include a copy of the manifest and an explanation of all efforts to locate the waste or manifest.

80) We selected answer B because:

EPA considers you a small quantity generator if your business produces more than 220 and less than 2,200 pounds (more than 100 and less than 1,000 kilograms) of hazardous waste in a calendar month. If you produce 1,000 kilograms or more of hazardous waste in any calendar month, or more than one kilogram of certain acutely hazardous wastes, you are subject to the more extensive regulations for large quantity generators. Large quantity generators may only store on site for a maximum of 90 days.

81) We selected answer A because:

According to 40 CFR 372, quantities that trigger reporting are 10,000 pounds of a toxic chemical used during the preceding calendar year.

82)   We selected answer D because:

On October 11, 1976, the federal government was given blanket authority by congress to regulate any substance that "may present an unreasonable risk of injury to health or the environment". Under the Toxic Substances Control Act the EPA has the responsibility to require manufacturers to test new chemicals entering the market stream to insure they do not pose an "unreasonable risk" to people or the environment. EPA can prohibit specified uses for a chemical or require or prohibit a specific means of disposal of a chemical. The law does not affect export to other countries.

83)   We selected answer B because:

Currently RCRA has two standards for determining if waste drums or containers are empty. For acutely hazardous waste, the drum must be: Triple rinsed using a solvent that will remove the waste; Washed in any manner that will achieve the same removal of waste as triple rinsing; Have the inner liner removed

84)   We selected answer B because:

This is the definition of radioactive half-life.

85)   We selected answer B because:

EPA must be notified at least **90 days** before a new chemical is manufactured. The other three answers are correct

86)   We selected answer D because:

Selection "A" is incorrect because OSHA requires powder-actuated tools to be inspected each day before loading (1926.302). Selection "B" should read 1000 psi to be accurate. Selection "C" is not correct because OSHA exempts concrete form cleaning from the 30 psi limitation.

87)   We selected answer D because:

There is not a category of protective footwear designed especially for Non-ionizing radiation workers. *Conductive footwear* offering a resistance below 450k OHMs is available to allow for dissipation of static charges. Typical applications would include some types of munitions manufacturing, cleaning tanks that have contained flammable liquids, etc. The *ANSI Std. Z41 "Safety-Toe Footwear"* groups Safety Toe Footwear into three classes which indicates the impact weight the shoes are designed to withstand while maintaining a 16/32 (15/32 for women) inch clearance inside the shoe. The classes are 75, 50 and 30. Electrical hazard shoes are designed to lessen the hazards of contact with electrical current. There are various special types of protective footwear that have extra protection from protruding nails, hot surfaces etc. Additionally, workers exposed during part of the day, to the hazards of very heavy objects, can wear foot caps. Foot caps are devices that fit over standard safety toed shoes or boots and protect the entire foot from the danger of falling objects.

88)   We selected answer B because:

Proper eye protection is among the most important safety precautions welders and metal cutters can take. The proper shade protection is very important to guard against the damage caused by UV and IR radiation created during these operations. The table below was taken directly from the OSHA standards additional information is contained in ANSI/ASC Z49.1-88.

OSHA 1926.102 Table E-2
FILTER LENS SHADE NUMBERS FOR PROTECTION AGAINST RADIANT ENERGY

Welding Operation	Shade Number
Shielded metal-arc welding 1/16, 3/32, 1/8, 5/32 inch diameter electrodes	10
Gas-shielded arc welding (nonferrous) 1/16, 3/32, 1/8, 5/32 inch diameter electrodes	11
Gas-shielded arc welding (ferrous) 1/16, 3/32, 1/8, 5/32 inch diameter electrodes	12
Shielded metal-arc welding 3/16, 7/32, 1/4 inch diameter electrodes	12
5/16, 3/8 inch diameter electrodes	14
Atomic hydrogen welding	10-14
Carbon-arc welding	14
Soldering	2
Torch brazing	3 or 4
Light cutting, up to 1 inch	3 or 4
Medium cutting, 1 inch to 6 inches	4 or 5
Heavy cutting, over 6 inches	5 or 6
Gas welding (light), up to 1/8 inch	4 or 5
Gas welding (medium), 1/8 inch to 1/2 inch	5 or 6
Gas welding (heavy), over 1/2 inch	6 or 8

89) We selected answer D because:

The most effective agents for Class B fires involving flammable liquids are Foam, CO_2, and Dry Chemical.

90) We selected answer A because:

For a belt and 6-foot lanyard a waist-height attachment would produce a 6-foot free fall.

91) We selected answer C because:

According to the National Safety Council's "Accident Prevention Manual for Industrial Operations." Tool rests should be adjusted to not more than 1/8 inch from the grinding wheel, tongue guards should be adjusted to 1/4 inch.

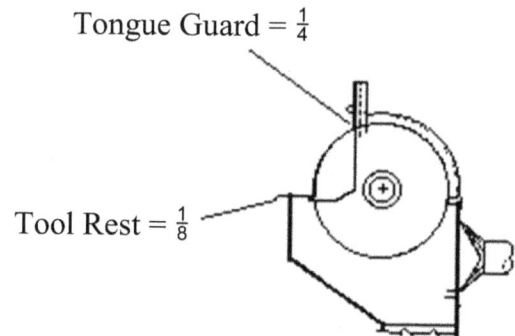

Tongue Guard = $\frac{1}{4}$

Tool Rest = $\frac{1}{8}$

92) We selected answer A because:

The standard hot wire combustible gas detector reads in percent LEL.

93) We selected answer D because:

According to OSHA at 1926.905 "Equipment shall not be operated within 50 feet of loaded holes". Selection "A" is not correct, drill holes should be large enough to freely admit the insertion of explosive cartridges. Selection "B" is in error, primers must never under any circumstance be tamped. In selection "C" the required distance is 50 feet.

94) We selected answer B because:

1926.800(g)(3) Designated person: At least one designated person shall be on duty above ground whenever any employee is working underground. This designated person shall be responsible for securing immediate aid and keeping an accurate count of employees underground in case of emergency. The designated person must not be so busy that the counting function is encumbered.

95) We selected answer A because:

Inspection of hoisting and rigging equipment before each job provides the greatest protection from use of defective equipment. Selection "B" is a good practice, however not as protective as choice "A". The frequency on selection "C" should be dependent on use, however in no case more than 12 months. Selection "D" is incorrect, bird-caged wire rope should be removed from service.

96) We selected answer D because:

Respirators may be used by more than one worker, however they must be cleaned and disinfected before use by another employee. They cannot simply be passed from person to person on a job site. All of the other selections are correct. Respirator users must be trained in the use and limitations of the apparatus. Respirators must be inspected at regular intervals and rescue equipment must be cleaned immediately after use so that the equipment is available should another emergency arise.

97) We selected answer A because:

OSHA 1926, Subpart P, Appendix B requires an excavation in Type A soil that is open less than 24 hours and is 12 feet or less in depth to have a maximum allowable slope of ½:1.

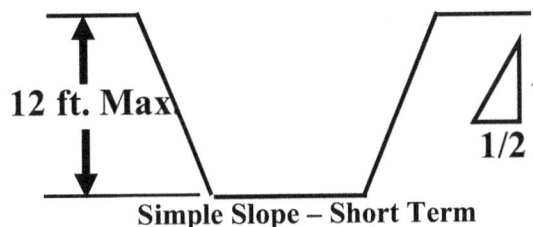

12 ft. Max

Simple Slope – Short Term

98) We selected answer D because:

A velometer is an instrument used to measure air velocity, often used in determining the airflow in ventilation systems. Selection "A", wind rose is a diagram showing the relative frequency and direction of wind loading. Selection "B", viscometer or viscosimeter is an instrument for determining the viscosity of slurries, fresh concrete, liquids etc. Selection "C", the westphal balance is a device used to measure the specific gravity of solids, minerals, liquids, etc.

99) We selected answer C because:
OSHA 1926, Subpart P, Appendix B requires an excavation in Type C soil that is 20 feet or less in depth to have a maximum allowable slope of 1½:1.

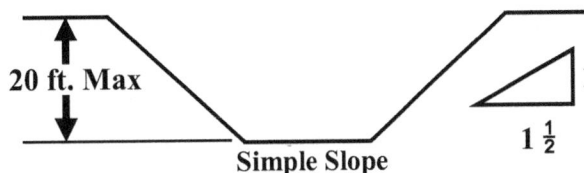

20 ft. Max

Simple Slope

100)   We selected answer B because:

Biological monitoring for uptake of lead can involve blood lead levels (PhB) and blood zinc protoporphyrin (ZPP), which can show recent uptake. Selection "A" would test for accumulations of carbon monoxide. Selection "C" is the biological marker for exposure to toluene. Selection "D" is a test for exposure to parathion.

Self-Assessment Exam Three Questions

1) On what frequency must self-contained breathing apparatus (SCBA) used as emergency or rescue equipment be inspected?

   A) Monthly.
   B) Annually.
   C) Semiannually.
   D) Weekly.

2) Which of the following would be the **best** use of direct reading instrumentation?

   A) To determine the amount of several different hazards.
   B) To monitor for sporadic increases in a particular contaminate.
   C) To provide generalizations about several different gases.
   D) To provide absolute accuracy during the ongoing assessment of confined spaces.

3) In which of the following conditions would the use of dilution ventilations be **most appropriate?**

   A) The source is very toxic.
   B) The source of contamination is a heavy particulate.
   C) Employees are in close contact with the source.
   D) The source of contamination is constant.

4) Field sanitation is a major concern on a construction site, of particular importance is the subject of drinking water. Accordingly, the rules concerning sanitation and drinking water are strict in the OSHA standards. All of the following describe specific requirements of an OSHA standard concerning potable water on a construction site **except?**

   A) Drinking from a common cup or from the lid on a water container is not allowed.
   B) All water containers must be marked and not used for any other purpose.
   C) Potable water must be available on the job site as soon as the foundation work is started.
   D) If single service cups are provided a dispenser and a disposal receptacle with a lid are required.

5) Which of the following symptoms would a person **not** experience when suffering from heatstroke?

    A) Loss of consciousness.
    B) Rapid temperature rise and hot dry skin.
    C) Severe headache.
    D) Profuse sweating and cool moist skin.

6) Toxic materials enter the body through which major routes?

    A) Inhalation, respiration, breathing.
    B) Inhalation, skin absorption, eating.
    C) Inhalation, skin absorption, ingestion.
    D) Inhalation, capillary absorption, intravenous.

7) In order of decreasing effectiveness, which of the following correctly indicates the order of corrective actions taken to prevent industrial dermatosis?

    A) Gloves, barrier cream, hygiene.
    B) Substitution, gloves, barrier cream.
    C) Gloves, hygiene, barrier cream.
    D) Substitution, hygiene, barrier cream, gloves.

8) Which of the following types of ionizing radiation is considered to be only an internal hazard?

    A) Neutron radiation.
    B) Beta radiation.
    C) Gamma or X-Ray.
    D) Alpha radiation.

9) Which of the following types of radiation from welding operations is the **most damaging** to the eye?

    A) Light.
    B) Ultraviolet.
    C) Infrared.
    D) Visible light.

10) If variations in noise levels are occurring at a rate more often than once per second, the noise is considered _____ under OSHA's noise standard.

    A) Impulse.
    B) Impact.
    C) Continuous.
    D) A and B above.

11) Which of the following heat stress indicators is **most commonly** used in the Health & Safety field?

    A) Wet Temperature Index.
    B) Dry Bulb and Globe Temperature Index.
    C) Skin Wettedness Index.
    D) Wet Bulb Globe Thermometer Index.

12) Which of the following diseases would you associate with the construction industry?

    A) Silicosis.
    B) Brucellosis.
    C) Anthrax.
    D) Raynaud's.

13) OSHA requires the use of a registered Professional Engineer (P.E.) to ensure the safety of complicated, unusual or high-risk structures. Which of the following fails to correctly identify a condition where OSHA requires the services of a registered professional engineer.

    A) To determine if an excavation is located far enough away from a building.
    B) To design frame scaffolds in excess of 125 ft in height.
    C) To design sloping and benching plans for excavations in type "C" soil deeper than 16 feet.
    D) To design personnel hoists in bridge tower construction.

14) Within the OSHA standards for construction, 1926.451 provides guidance on the requirements and specifications for various types of scaffolds. Among the requirement are several specifications concerning the type and use of wooden planking. All of the following are requirements from OSHA 1926.451 **except?**

    A) Scaffold planking must be at least 1,500 psi fiber (stress grade).
    B) Scaffold planking shall be Scaffold Grade or equivalent.
    C) On a light duty scaffold (25 psf) the maximum permissible span for 2 × 10 nominal thickness lumber is 8 feet.
    D) Bricks or cinder blocks are permissible for mud sills.

15) Which of the following descriptions **best** fits the intent of the OSHA standards when referring to a "Competent Person"?

    A) The person who has the authority to shut down the operation anytime the risk analysis indicates that a moderate or greater hazard is reasonably expected to cause injury to workers.
    B) The person who is capable of identifying existing and predictable hazards in the surroundings or working conditions which are unsanitary, hazardous, or dangerous to employees, and who has authorization to take prompt corrective measures to eliminate them.
    C) The person required at confined space, and hoisting & rigging, and excavation & trenching job sites.
    D) The supervisor with the ability of identifying existing and future hazards on the job site and who reports directly to the person who has responsible charge of the operation.

16) According to OSHA, what spacing is required between the required ladders in excavations classified as trenched?

    A) 50 feet.
    B) 100 feet.
    C) 10 feet.
    D) 30 feet.

17) The OSHA regulation covering underground construction is 1926.800, which covers the construction of underground tunnels, shafts, chambers and cut-and-cover excavations. According to OSHA 1926.800 ventilation must be provided to maintain underground air quality. How many cubic feet of fresh air is required for each worker underground?

   A) 50 ft^3
   B) 100 ft^3
   C) 400 ft^3
   D) 200 ft^3

18) The physiological property of matter that defines the capacity of a chemical to harm or injure a living organism by other than mechanical means is the definition of?

   A) Injury.
   B) Illness.
   C) Toxicity.
   D) Hazard.

19) Within the OSHA standards for construction, 1926.451 provides guidance on the requirements and specifications for various types of scaffolds. According to this standard all of the following are correct **except?**
   A) Scaffold erection is not permitted except under the direction of a competent person.
   B) Guardrails and toeboards shall be installed on all open sides and ends of platforms more than 10 feet above the ground or floor, except needle beam scaffolds and floats.
   C) All planking used must be scaffold grade or equivalent.
   D) Scaffolds must be built with a safety factor of 5.

20) Depending on the industry, frequent inspection of chains is required, the **best** way to inspect chains during these inspections is to:

   A) Perform a detailed link-by-link inspection of entire chain.
   B) Check links with a caliper and compare at least 10 links.
   C) Compare twist on end sections.
   D) Check for cracks in end links.

21) Which of the following electrical devices would **most likely** contain polychlorinated biphenyl (PCBs)?

A) Circuit breakers, panel board and Unistrut.
B) Transformers, capacitors, fluorescent light ballasts.
C) Fuses, wiring and meters.
D) Meters, relays and switches.

22) The OSHA regulation covering underground construction is 1926.800, which covers the construction of underground tunnels, shafts, chambers and cut-and-cover excavations. The regulation establishes a "competent person" as the responsible party for various inspection and oversight operations in the underground environment. Which of the following is **not** a specific duty of a competent person according to 1910.800?

A) Inspection of all hauling equipment prior to each shift.
B) Inspection of all drilling equipment prior to each use.
C) Inspection of barricades used to seal off unused headings.
D) Inspection of the work area for ground stability.

23) The OSHA regulation covering underground construction is 1926.800, which covers the construction of underground tunnels, shafts, chambers and cut-and-cover excavations. Under the provisions of the standard employees must be taught to recognize and avoid hazards associated with underground construction. Which of the following is **not** required by OSHA 1926.800 to be included in the training provided employees working underground?

A) Sanitation.
B) Air monitoring.
C) Flood control.
D) Check-in and check-out procedures.

24) Which of the following correctly indicates the minimum access width leading to an exit required by the NFPA "Life Safety Code"?

A) 32 inches.
B) 22 inches.
C) 28 inches.
D) 36 inches.

25) Which of the following is **not** included in the qualifications OSHA has established for blasters?

   A) Must be able to read and write.
   B) Knowledge and competency in the use of each type of blasting method to be used on the job.
   C) Good physical condition.
   D) Possession of a state blasters license.

26) The hoods on grinders and cutting wheels establish the platform for a tongue guard that must be placed within 1/4 inch of the periphery of the wheel at all times. The hood also serves several other purposes including:

   A) Covering at least 85% of the wheel.
   B) Removal of dust and dirt generated by the operation.
   C) Providing protection from falling into the wheel.
   D) Removal of particles and shielding operator from hazard if wheel should break.

27) What is the primary reason for Safety and Health accident investigation?

   A) To establish who or what was at fault.
   B) To establish a baseline for further analysis.
   C) To determine the facts surrounding the event.
   D) To determine the obvious cause factors.

28) All of the instruments could be used to measure the radiation from an industrial X-Ray machine **except?**

   A) Geiger Counter.
   B) Cutie pie.
   C) Condenser R-meters.
   D) Scatter Absorbers.

29) Concentrations of gases and vapors are commonly expressed as?

   A) Parts per million by weight.
   B) Parts per million by volume.
   C) mg per cubic centimeter.
   D) mg per square meter.

30) During a forklift operation, you observe the back of a forklift tip as a heavy load is being lifted. Which of the following is the proper course of action?

    A) Add extra counter weight to stabilize the operation until the load can be lifted without tipping.
    B) Tip the mast back once the load is lifted this will shift the weight to the rear and the forktruck will level itself.
    C) Add air to the load side tires which will raise that end.
    D) Do not continue with this lift.

31) Entry into a confined space is required at one of your construction sites. The oxygen concentration in the confined space has been measured at 16%. Which of the following **most correctly** indicates the danger to personnel entering this atmosphere?

    A) 16% oxygen causes tingling in the fingers and toes.
    B) This level of oxygen is adequate for rescue operations only.
    C) Time spent in this atmosphere should be limited, if a worker experiences blue lips they should be removed.
    D) This level of oxygen could cause impairment of judgment and difficult breathing.

32) The horizontal grouping of elements in the periodic table is called a _____?

    A) Tribe.
    B) Period.
    C) Group or Family.
    D) Element.

33) The atomic number of an element indicates the total number of?

    A) Neutrons.
    B) Protons.
    C) Protons and Neutrons.
    D) Electrons.

34) A liquid with a flash point of 100°F and a boiling point of 110°F would be classified by the OSHA and the NFPA as a:

    A) Class I flammable liquid.
    B) Class IA combustible liquid.
    C) Class IB flammable liquid.
    D) Class II combustible liquid.

35) Sound Pressure Levels are measured in which of the following units?

    A) Dynes per cm^3
    B) Millibars.
    C) Microns (micrometers).
    D) Microbars.

36) According to OSHA at 1910.147 an energy control program is required to ensure that before any worker performs servicing/maintenance on a machine or equipment, where the unexpected startup or release of stored energy could occur and cause injury, the machine or equipment shall be isolated from the energy source. This generally requires a physical lock and tag arrangement to meet the intent of the OSHA. When is it permissible to only use a tagout system of protection?

    A) If locks cost more than tags.
    B) On overlapping shift work.
    C) When other protective measures are in place.
    D) When the point of operation is higher than 7 feet above floor level.

37) When placing a standard straight ladder the horizontal distance from the base to the vertical plane of the support should be approximately _____ the ladder length between supports.

    A) 1/3.
    B) 1/4.
    C) 1/2.
    D) 1/8.

38) In the practice of Safety and Health, training is often offered as a universal solution. However, safety and health training should be targeted to real problems. Training should only be recommended as the solution to problems where increased knowledge or skill is needed or where required by directive. Which of the following **best** describes the reason or objective for after training testing?

    A) To weed out weak performers.
    B) To spot workers who have "attitude" problems.
    C) To spot weaknesses in the training program.
    D) To allow the students to see how much they learned.

39) What is the molecular weight of dry air?

    A) 30.
    B) 45.
    C) 1.
    D) 90.

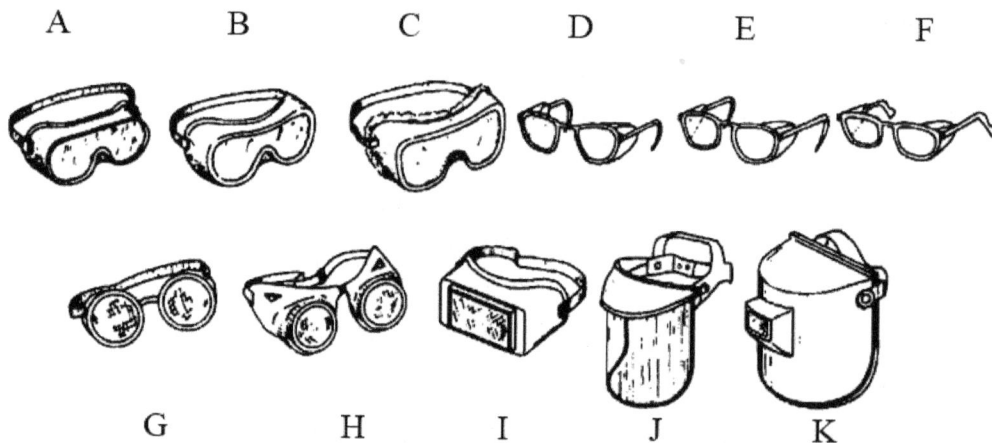

40) Using the illustration shown above which personal protective equipment would provide the greatest degree of protection and be the most appropriate for a worker transporting or handling H_2SO_4?

    A) A & K.
    B) C and J.
    C) C & D.
    D) J or K.

41) Which of the following definitions is correct? Specific gravity of a liquid is _____.

A) Equal to the density.
B) Mass per unit volume of substance.
C) Ratio of wt. of volume to wt. of equal volume of water.
D) Ratio of wt. of volume to wt. of an equal volume of hydrogen.

42) Which of the following does **not** require an equipment grounding conductor?

A) A double reverse delta electrical system.
B) A double insulated hand tool.
C) A circuit that is protected with circuit breakers.
D) A system with a wye connected transformer.

43) Which of the following poses the **most common** exposure to ultraviolet radiation?

A) Stick welding.
B) Black Light.
C) Direct Sunlight.
D) Sun Guns.

44) While monitoring plant workers you discover that the TLV-STEL is being exceeded, for more than one hour, each work shift. Which of the following courses of action is appropriate?

A) Continue monitoring and compute a new TWA.
B) Recommend that the operation be curtailed immediately.
C) Send the instrumentation for calibration.
D) Continue as long as you do not exceed TLV-C values.

45) Which of the following conditions provides the **best** opportunity for obtaining a precise reading of colorimetric tubes?

A) Fluorescent lighting of at least 150-foot candles.
B) Daylight or incandescent lighting.
C) Mercury vapor lighting.
D) A 10,000-watt sun gun.

46) The specific gravity of water is?

    A) 1.1 to 1.
    B) 5 to 1.
    C) 1.
    D) 5.

47) When using a solid sorbent tube for personal sampling which of the following would be considered the **most important?**

    A) Place the tube in the breathing zone.
    B) Spike blanks to check the laboratory QC.
    C) Ship bulk samples in a separate package.
    D) Use plastic caps instead of tape to seal tube at end of sampling.

48) Which of the following **best** describes the effect of carbon monoxide on the blood?

    A) Replaces oxygen and reduces white blood cells.
    B) Replaces oxygen and reduces transportation of oxygen.
    C) Reduces oxygen capacity of lungs.
    D) Reduces oxygen in lungs and causes edema.

49) Which of the following **best** describes the greatest single error in colorimetric sampling devices?

    A) Gel coagulation.
    B) Temperature extremes.
    C) Pump airflow inaccuracy.
    D) Interferences by other contaminants.

50) Which of the following **best** defines grab sampling?

    A) Cheapest of all methods.
    B) Instantaneous sample.
    C) Very complex.
    D) Always taken in the breathing zone.

51) Guarding of power transmission parts involves the principle of covering all moving parts in such a manner that no part of the body can come in contact with a moving part. Generally moving parts _____ or less from the floor must be guarded?

    A) 8 feet.
    B) 7 feet.
    C) 10 feet.
    D) 9 feet.

52) In industrial environments the concept of local exhaust ventilation is used extensively. The purpose of local exhaust ventilation is to:

    A) Prevent any entrance of air contaminants.
    B) Remove contaminants at their source.
    C) Provide dilution ventilation.
    D) Provide spot ventilation for comfort.

53) Which of the following is **not** a requirement for a flammable liquid "Safety" can?

    A) Spring loaded cover that opens at 5 psi.
    B) Flame arrestor.
    C) Fusible link.
    D) Metal construction.

54) Which of the following correctly indicates the lowest percentage of oxygen allowed by OHSA at ambient pressure?

    A) 16.5%.
    B) 19%.
    C) 19.5%.
    D) 20%.

55) During an OSHA inspection of your site, who determines what areas will be visited and for how long?

    A) The OSHA Compliance Officer.
    B) The employee representative.
    C) A Certified Health & Safety Technician.
    D) The owner.

56) Often when an OSHA Compliance Safety & Health Officer (CSHO) arrives at the construction site for an inspection a management official or safety engineer is not available to accompany them on the inspection. Normally the CSHO will wait for you a reasonable amount of time before beginning the inspection. Which of the following **best** describes the OSHA definition of a reasonable amount of time?

A) One hour.
B) 15 minutes.
C) One hour and a half.
D) Two hours.

57) During an OSHA inspection of your worksite the union steward has requested from the OSHA Compliance Safety & Health Officer (CSHO), a separate in-briefing (opening conference) so that they can talk without management representatives interfering. Will the CSHO conduct a separate opening conference for the union representatives?

A) No, strictly prohibited.
B) No, but the CSHO will allow them to write down any additional information they think he/she should know.
C) Yes, as per OSHA policy the CSHO will conduct two opening conferences.
D) Yes, but not until after the inspection is complete.

58) Which of the following statements is **not** correct concerning the conduct of an OSHA Compliance Safety & Health Officer (CSHO) during a programmed inspection of your jobsite?

A) The CSHO can provide assistance to you in determining how to abate violations.
B) The CSHO can order the men off of a job if he uncovers a imminent danger situation.
C) The CSHO can conduct a second closing conference by telephone if they cannot get it all done at the first one.
D) The CSHO can defer an inspection during a strike or labor dispute.

59) Section 17(k) of the OSHAct explains that a serious violation is, ". . . a serious violation shall be deemed to exist in a place of employment if there is a substantial probability that death or serious physical harm could result from a condition which exists, or from one or more practices, means, methods, operations, or processes which have been adopted or are in use, in such place of employment unless the employer did not, and could not with the exercise of reasonable diligence, know of the presence of the violation." In determining if a serious violation exists, the CSHO finds that the supervisor had full knowledge of the hazard. Does this knowledge constitute a serious violation?

    A) No, the supervisor is considered an employee not the employer.
    B) Yes, the supervisor represents the employer and a supervisor's knowledge of the hazard amounts to employer knowledge.
    C) No, the supervisor could have chosen not to have told the owner.
    D) Yes, the owner should have known if he would have been doing his job.

60) Which of the following is true concerning explosive equipment? Explosive proof equipment is allowed to operate in a flammable or explosive atmosphere because it is capable of:

    A) Containing internal explosions.
    B) Not producing sparks under any condition.
    C) Operating below the auto ignition temperature.
    D) Shutting down the equipment serviced in an emergency.

61) On multi-employer worksites implementation of the OSHA Hazard Communication Program poses some additional concerns. If the general contractor handles or uses hazardous chemicals in such a manner that sub-contract employees working on the site may be exposed then the general contractor is required do all of the following **except?**

    A) Provide the sub with the details of the labeling system used in the workplace.
    B) Provide the sub with a MSDS or notify the sub where the MSDSs are centrally located for each hazardous material they may be exposed to while working on site.
    C) Rewrite the sub-contractors operating procedures for all foreseeable emergency situations.
    D) Provide training to the sub-contractor for any precautionary measures that need to be taken to protect employees during the

workplace's normal operating conditions.

62) Which of the following would **not** require a label under the provisions of OSHA 1926.59, Hazard Communication standard?

    A) Compressed gas cylinders.
    B) A small container used to dispense chemicals by workers at the jobsite.
    C) A storage tank of hazardous chemicals.
    D) Fuel tank in a pickup truck at construction site.

63) The requirements for lift-slab operations are very stringent and operations receive a lot of attention from OSHA because of the potential for large accidental loss. All lift-slab operations must be designed and planned by a registered professional engineer (P.E.). After the slab is lifted into position by jacks/lifting units, the slab can be positively secured to the building columns. All welding must be done by certified welders familiar with the plans and specifications for the lift-slab operation. Transfer of weight from the jacks to the building support columns cannot take place until the welds on the shear plates have achieved maximum strength. Accordingly, the weight cannot be transferred until?

    A) The welds have cooled for 30 minutes.
    B) The welds have cooled for 5 minutes.
    C) The welds have cooled to 120 degrees.
    D) The welds have cooled to air temperature.

64) In which case should an electrical branch circuit be protected by a Ground Fault Circuit Interrupter (GFCI)?

    A) When used in a industrial environment.
    B) If extremely long extension cords are normally used.
    C) Adjacent to wet locations such as swimming pools.
    D) In all outside locations.

65) Which of the following is true concerning electrically operated hand held power tools on the construction site?

    A) All power tools must be grounded.
    B) Double and triple insulated tools do not need to be grounded.
    C) Power operated tools must be connected to a GFCI when used outdoors.
    D) GFCIs are required on construction sites.

66) Which of the following sound frequency ranges is generally considered to be the most harmful to hearing, especially the speech range?

    A) 37.5- 500 Hz.
    B) 1000-4000 Hz.
    C) 8000-16000 Hz.
    D) 16000-32000 Hz.

67) Which of the following groups of hydrocarbons would have the **greatest** chance of not being flammable?

    A) Aliphatic Hydrocarbons.
    B) Aromatic Hydrocarbons.
    C) Halogenated Hydrocarbons.
    D) Ethers.

68) A welding operator using argon for shielding gas would **most likely** be welding which of the following materials?

    A) Tungsten.
    B) Galvanized Steel.
    C) Copper.
    D) Aluminum.

69) Traditional open frame safety glasses would be **least effective** in protecting an employee's eyes in which of the following situations?

    A) Chipping rock.
    B) Pouring molten metals.
    C) Working in a high concentration of acid.
    D) Sharpening tools at a stand grinder.

70) What type of electrical equipment is required in a spray paint booth?

    A) NEC Class I, Div 2.
    B) NEC Class I, Div 1.
    C) NEC Class II, Div 2.
    D) NEC Class III, Div 1.

71) When is the use of a Gas Mask permissible in an atmosphere that is Immediately Dangerous to Life or Health due to the presence of a toxic contaminant?

    A) Never.
    B) When it is used for escape only.
    C) As a backup measure.
    D) When SCBA is being inspected.

72) The principle of guarding indicating Zero Mechanical State is generally understood to mean?

    A) All energy sources are powered down.
    B) All electrical energy is off.
    C) Guards are in a zero or down position.
    D) The machine is not operational (Zero Mechanical State).

73) Seat belts are required to be worn when operating a forklift?

    A) True.
    B) False.
    C) False, if the forklift is equipped with roll over protection.
    D) True, if the forklift is equipped with roll over protection.

74) In accordance with the Process Safety Management standard, who is responsible for contract employee training?

    A) Employee.
    B) Prime contractor.
    C) Contract employer.
    D) OSHA & the contract employer.

75) Which of the following is a widely used quick screening test to determine the potential of a chemical to be a carcinogen?
    A) Ames Assay.
    B) Soot bio-assay.
    C) Pyrolysis.
    D) Precipitation.

76) Any employee engaged in a steel erection activity who is on a walking/working surface with an unprotected side or edge more than ____ feet (4.6m) above a lower level shall be protected from fall hazards by guardrail systems, safety net systems, personal fall arrest systems, positioning device systems or fall restraint systems.
    A) 6.
    B) 10.
    C) 15.
    D) 20.

77) The **simplest** and **most effective** way to display data to get an instant picture is the use of the?
    A) Line chart.
    B) Bar chart.
    C) Pie chart.
    D) Area chart.

78) In some combustible gas meters an electrical circuit called the wheatstone bridge circuit is used to measure the mixture of combustible gas to air. Which of the following characteristics concerning this balanced bridge circuit is **not** true?
    A) The presence of a combustible mixture causes catalytic combustion decreasing resistance shown as meter movement.
    B) One leg of the circuit is called a hot wire.
    C) The platinum element can be poisoned by small amounts of silicone.
    D) The hot wire detector requires oxygen to function.

79) Which article of the National Electrical Code deals with hazardous locations?
    A) Article 407.
    B) Article 101.
    C) Article 20.
    D) Article 500.

80) The Safety Data Sheet (SDS) must contain all of the following **except?**
 A) Fire and explosion data.
 B) Health Hazard data.
 C) Protective equipment requirements.
 D) Manufacturer's part number.

81) According to the Fire Protection Handbook®, all of the following are important steps in examining the scene of a fire **except?**
 A) Take as many photographs as possible.
 B) Contact the insurance company.
 C) Check the fire suppression system.
 D) Interview the fire department responders.

82) What is the first step when doing CPR?
 A) Check airway.
 B) Check breathing.
 C) Check circulation.
 D) Start chest thrusts.

83) 40CFR264 requires that the generators of hazardous waste must do all of the following **except?**
 A) Develop a written schedule for inspecting monitoring equipment, safety and emergency equipment, security devices and operating and structural equipment.
 B) Develop a contingency plan that describes the actions that facility personnel must take in case of fire, explosions or unplanned releases of hazardous waste.
 C) Make arrangements with the local fire, police and emergency teams to ensure their awareness and that they can respond within 10 minutes of notification.
 D) Develop a waste analysis plan that describes the details for analyzing each type of hazardous waste.

84) The possibility of fire during construction operations is higher than during regular occupancy. Accordingly, storage of flammable liquid materials is strictly controlled on a construction site. Which of the following **best** describes the correct safety practices concerning storage of flammable/combustible liquids in a building under construction.
- A) Flammables stored inside not in an approved flammable storage cabinet are limited to 10 gallons.
- B) Flammables stored inside not in an approved flammable storage cabinet are limited to 25 gallons.
- C) Stairwell storage is limited to 60 gallons of flammables and 120 gallons of combustibles.
- D) Flammables cannot be stored on a construction site at any time, combustibles are limited to 10 gallons or a one-day supply whichever is less.

85) An employee who has experienced a significant threshold shift (STS) is currently working in an area where the Time Weighted Average (TWA) noise level is 100 dBA. If hearing protection is used as the control method, how much attenuation must be provided by the hearing protectors?
- A) 10 dB.
- B) 5 dB.
- C) 20 dB.
- D) 15 dB.

86) The requirements for an Assured Equipment Grounding Conductor Program are contained in 29 CFR 1926.404. This standard requires a written description of the employer's assured equipment grounding conduction program, including the specific procedures to be used, be kept at the jobsite. Additionally, testing must be done to determine the continuity of the equipment grounding conductor and to ensure the correct polarity of receptacles and plugs. Which of the following items of test equipment would be the **most accurate** in measuring the amount of resistance in an equipment ground?
- A) Lamp and battery.
- B) Battery and buzzer/bell.
- C) Neon lamp.
- D) Ground loop impedance tester.

87) Which of the following provides the **best** definition of Standard Threshold Shift according to OSHA?
    A) An average change in hearing threshold of 5 dB or more at 500, 1000 & 3000 Hz.
    B) An average change in hearing threshold of 10 dB or more at 2000, 3000 & 4000 Hz.
    C) An average change in hearing threshold of 15 dB or more at 500, 3000 & 6000 Hz.
    D) An average change in hearing threshold of 20 dB or more at 2000, 3000 & 4000 Hz.

88) The medical questionnaire that is required when you place an employee in your respiratory protection must be evaluated by?
    A) The industrial hygienist.
    B) The safety director.
    C) A licensed health care professional.
    D) Any supervisor in the employee's chain.

89) When taking noise measurements in a non-reverberant environment, instructions often call for placing the microphone in the workers hearing zone. Which of the following **best** describes the hearing zone?
    A) An area surrounding the body for a distance of 12 inches.
    B) A hemisphere 9-18 inches in radius and centered on the shoulder.
    C) A hemisphere 6-9 inches in radius and forward of the shoulders.
    D) A sphere 2 feet in diameter centered on the head.

90) Which of the following is **not** true concerning the electrical Ground Fault Circuit Interrupter?
    A) It requires an equipment ground to function.
    B) It is a very fast acting device.
    C) It will not detect line-to-line faults.
    D) It is designed for personnel protection.

91) According to OSHA exposure to impulsive or impact noise should not exceed _____ peak sound pressure level?
    A) 130 dB.
    B) 115 dB.
    C) 110 dB.
    D) 140 dB.

92) One of the problems associated with arc welding of stainless steel is the production of aerosols containing:
   A) Nickel and Chromium.
   B) Carbon and Nickel.
   C) Fluorides, Nickel and Chromium.
   D) Copper, Nickel and Acid gases.

93) In developing a safety training program, the **most essential** consideration is:
   A) Training staff.
   B) Training methods.
   C) Content of training program.
   D) Training objectives.

94) A direct reading instrument indicates a concentration of 2.5% for a hazardous material that has a Permissible Exposure Limit (PEL) of 250 ppm and an Immediately Dangerous to Life and Health (IDLH) of 2500 ppm and a Lower Explosive Limit (LEL) of 25,000 ppm. You have been assigned the task of respirator selection for entry into this atmosphere. Which of the following statements is the **most correct?**
   A) The instrument shows a reading in excess of the PEL and IDLH.
   B) The instrument shows a reading below the PEL, IDLH and LEL.
   C) The direct reading instrument indicates a concentration below the LEL but above the IDLH and PEL.
   D) The instrument shows a reading equal to the LEL, which is above the IDLH and PEL.

95) Which of the following trades would **most likely** be exposed to the damaging effects of fluorides?
   A) Welder.
   B) Stone Mason.
   C) Laborer.
   D) Carpenter.

96) Which of the following **best** fits the description of an anti-two block device?
   A) A device installed on an overhead crane to prevent lifting a weight beyond the load limit.
   B) A device designed to keep safety blocks from being inserted into a power press ram control.
   C) A device to prevent over travel of the load block on a mobile crane.
   D) A device that limits the amount of material that can be deposited in the muck bucket attachment on a hoist-way man-basket.

97) Which of the following statements would be correct concerning the stacking of bricks?
   A) Bricks must not be stacked over 8 feet in height.
   B) Bricks must not be stacked over 6 feet in height.
   C) Brick stacks must be tapered back 1½ inches in every foot of height above the 3-foot level.
   D) Brick stacks must be tapered back 2 inches in every foot of height above the 4-foot level.

98) Which of the following is the **most correct** concerning the maintenance of training records required by the OSHA Hazard Communication Standard?
   A) Training records must be maintained by the employee.
   B) Training records must be maintained by the employer.
   C) Training records must be maintained at the worksite.
   D) There is no requirement in OSHA to maintain worker training records.

99) Each employee on a scaffold more than _____ feet above a lower level shall be provided with fall protection to prevent from falling to that lower level.
   A) 3.
   B) 6.
   C) 10.
   D) 12.

100) Which of the following refers to the process of bonding a flammable liquid dispensing can?

A) Connecting the can to a grounding rod.
B) Connecting the can to a grounding strap.
C) Connecting the can to the equipment ground.
D) Connecting the can to other conductive objects.

Self-Assessment Exam Three Answers

1) We selected answer A because:

OSHA requires monthly inspections for self-contained breathing apparatus.

2) We selected answer B because:

Direct reading instrumentation is a very broad category and range from detector tubes to portable gas chromatographs that are capable of detecting just about every chemical one could encounter. Additionally, direct reading instrumentation can be very accurate or, in the case of detector tubes, not so accurate. However, direct reading instrumentation does suffer from one common ailment, almost all of these instruments suffer from interference by other contaminants.

3) We selected answer D because:

Dilution ventilation is the preferred solution when relatively non-toxic emissions are produced, when the source is mainly gases or vapors (not primarily heavy particulates) and when employees do not work in the immediate vicinity or direct path of the emission source. The old adage "no pollution through more dilution" is often very appropriate, however when toxic, heavy, direct path, time inconsistent, or large sources of emissions are encountered, the solution is point source removal through local exhaust ventilation.

4) We selected answer C because:

OSHA requires all job sites have an adequate supply of potable water. This includes the "dirt work" phase of construction through installation of sanitary facilities. OSHA 1926.51 states

- "An adequate supply of potable water shall be provided in all places of employment.
- Portable containers used to dispense drinking water shall be capable of being tightly closed, and equipped with a tap. Water shall not be dipped from containers.
- Any container used to distribute drinking water shall be clearly marked as to the nature of its contents and not be used for any

other purpose.
- The common drinking cup is prohibited.
- Where single service cups (to be used but once) are supplied, both sanitary container for the unused cups and a receptacle for disposing of the used cups shall be provided."

5) We selected answer D because:

During heatstroke (sunstroke) the body temperature rises and reaches a point where the heat-regulating mechanism breaks down completely. The body temperature then rises rapidly. The symptoms are hot dry skin, severe headache, visual disturbances, rapid temperature rise, and loss of consciousness.

6) We selected answer C because:

The most common ways for toxic materials to enter the body is through the skin by absorption, by inhalation and through ingestion.

7) We selected answer B because:

It is generally accepted within the safety and health industry that substitution is the most effective control method for the prevention of industrial dermatosis. Substitution is followed by gloves and barrier cream. Good hygiene practice is, of course, required in all industrial settings.

8) We selected answer D because:

Alpha radiation is non-penetrating and is not considered an external hazard because of the protection provided by the outer layer of skin. Note - in this instance the eyes are considered an internal exposure.

9) We selected answer C because:

Both Ultraviolet (UV) and Infrared radiation (IR) will cause damage to the eye. However, IR is very penetrating and passes through the cornea to the retina of the eye causing permanent damage. Ultraviolet radiation will cause eye burn (Arc Eye) that is painful and disabling but usually the signs and symptoms disappear in 12 to 36 hours and, as stated earlier, are confined to the cornea.

10) We selected answer C because:

If the occurrence of the sound is greater than once per second the sound is considered to be continuous and should be measured as continuous sound. Ref. OSHA 29 CFR 1910.95.

11) We selected answer D because:

The most commonly used heat stress index is the National Institute for Occupational Safety and Health (NIOSH) Wet Bulb Globe Thermometer Index (WBGT).

12) We selected answer D because:

Brucellosis is an infection caused by drinking unpasteurized milk. *Anthrax* is a bacterial infection from animals. *Silicosis* is a *Pneumoconiosis* of quartz miners. A combination of cold and vibration causes Raynaud's phenomenon. This is a condition of the fingers and hands characterized by pallor caused by a diminished blood supply. The disease is most prevalent among workers who use vibrating machinery and are exposed to the cold. Many construction workers encounter these conditions.

13) We selected answer C because:

There is continuing controversy over the use of the terms registered professional engineer, professional engineer, a component engineer etc. within the OSHA directives. OSHA has promised standardization in the near future for the "Professional Engineer" requirement and a raft of other misused or undefined terms, eg: certified, competent, qualified, highly qualified, registered etc. However, according to the current OSHA standards selection "A" is correct. 1926.651 requires a P.E. determine if an excavation will affect adjacent structures. Selection "B" is also correct 1926.451(d)(9) requires the services of a P.E. in designing frame scaffolds in excess of 125 feet in height. Selection "C" is not correct, the P.E. is only required to be involved if the excavation is at a depth of 20 feet or greater. Selection "D" is correct and can be found at 1926.552(c)(17)(i).

14) We selected answer D because:

OSHA at 1926.451 provides specific guidance concerning scaffolding. A good review of this section is in order prior to taking the CHST examination. Selection "A" is correct, scaffold planking must

MATERIAL					
	Full thickness undressed lumber			Nominal Thickness Lumber	
Working load (psf)	25	50	75	25	50
Permissible span (ft)	10	8	6	8	6

be at least 1500 psi fiber (Stress Grade) scaffold grade lumber. This 1500 psi fiber refers to the strength of the lumber in bending. Selection "B" is correct. Selection "C" is also correct, OSHA offers this chart from which to select spans.

Selection "D" is obviously incorrect, the sill and base plate is a very important part of the overall scaffold foundation. Often the base plate cannot distribute the high loads from the scaffold adequately, in this case a timber sill is required. The sill provides a friction surface and spreads loads over a larger area then the base plate. Sills are most often wood, but come in many different sizes depending on the loads involved. Often a 2 × 10 wood sill is used, it should be continuous and should be centered under the leg so as to support at least two legs. Obviously, bricks or cement blocks are just not adequate and are prohibited by OSHA.

15) We selected answer B because:

OSHA defines a competent person as "one who is capable of identifying existing and predictable hazards in the surroundings or working conditions which are unsanitary, hazardous, or dangerous to employees, and who has authorization to take prompt corrective measures to eliminate them". Additionally, the competent person should be a person who has extensive knowledge/experience in a particular activity or job function.

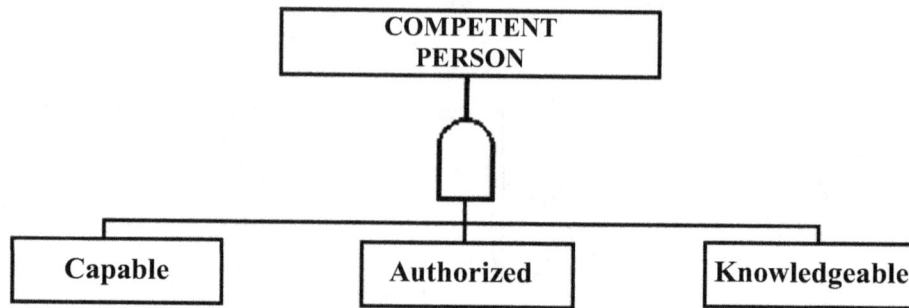

The result is a system fed by an "and" gate. The competent person must be capable "and" authorized "and" knowledgeable. Failure of any one of the elements results in a failure of the entire system.

16) We selected answer A because:

Means of egress from trench excavations such as a stairway, ladder, ramp or other safe means of egress are required in trench excavations that are 4 feet or more in depth and located so as to require **no more than 25 feet of lateral travel** for workers. Ladders placed every 50 running feet of trench would provide a maximum of 25 feet of travel in each direction, assuming a initial ladder at the start of the trench run. OSHA 1926.651.

17) We selected answer D because:

To prevent any dangerous or harmful accumulation of dusts, fumes, mists, vapors, or gases OSHA 1926.800(k)(1)(ii)(2) requires a minimum of 200 cubic feet of fresh air per minute to be supplied for each employee underground.

18) We selected answer C because:

The question accurately states the definition of toxicity.

19) We selected answer D because:

OSHA 1926.451 requires all scaffolds and their components to be capable of supporting without failure at least 4 times the maximum intended load. Safety factor is defined as:

$$\frac{\text{Maximum load}}{\text{Breaking strength}} = SafetyFactor$$

Or stated another way, with a safety factor of four the maximum allowable load will never be greater than 25% of the load it takes to cause the scaffold to fail. Safety factors are developed to allow for greater than anticipated:

- Loads (extra men, equipment etc.)
- Wind loading
- Faulty and defective equipment
- Poor scaffold design

20) We selected answer A because:

Chain inspections should be done visually in an attempt to detect any elongation or other defect. This is best accomplished by a link-by-link inspection. Overall measurements or caliper readings of a section are often misleading because not all links will be affected or damaged.

21) We selected answer B because:

Polychlorinated biphenyl (PCBs) are found in certain electrical devices such as transformers, capacitors, fluorescent light ballasts, etc., as well as in heat transfer enclosures and investment casting waxes in foundries. In 1978 EPA banned the use of PCB in light ballasts, capacitors and transformers, however it is still possible to find equipment containing PCBs.

22) We selected answer C because:

In accordance with OSHA 1926.800 a competent person is responsible for:

- Air monitoring
- Testing the atmosphere for flammable limits before restoring power and equipment and before returning to work after a ventilation system has been shut down due to hazardous levels of flammable gas or methane
- Inspection of the work area for ground stability
- Inspection of all drilling equipment prior to each use
- Inspection of all hauling equipment before each shift
- Visually checking all hoisting machinery, equipment, anchorages, and rope at the beginning of each shift and during hoisting if necessary

The inspection of barricaded headings is not specifically covered in the OSHA directives.

23) We selected answer A because:

OSHA 1926.800 requires that employees be taught to recognize and avoid hazards associated with underground construction. The instruction should include:

- Air monitoring
- Illumination
- Flood Control equipment
- Personal Protective Equipment
- Fire Prevention & Protection
- Emergency procedures including evacuation plans and check-in and check-out systems

- Ventilation
- Communications
- Mechanical

- Explosives

Sanitation is not specifically included in the OSHA standard.

24) We selected answer C because:

The minimum access to an exit required by NFPA 101 the "Life Safety Code" is 28 inches.

25) We selected answer D because:

Federal OSHA does not specifically require a state blasters license, although the state you are operating in may very well have such a requirement. OSHA does require that a blaster:

- Be able to understand and give written and oral orders
- Shall be in good physical condition and not be addicted to narcotics, intoxicants, or similar types of drugs
- Shall be qualified, by reason of training, knowledge, or experience, in the field of transporting, storing, handling, and use of explosives, and have a working knowledge of State and local laws and regulations which pertain to explosives

26) We selected answer D because:

Hoods on grinding and cutting operations serve a dual function; they protect the worker from the hazards of a bursting wheel, and provide for removal of the dirt, dust and material generated during grinding or cutting operations.

27) We selected answer C because:

According to the National Safety Council accident investigation should be conducted to provide the facts, if fault-finding is attempted the investigation may cause more harm than good. Mishap investigation is conducted to determine both obvious and hidden cause factors. It does tend to serve as the baseline for further analysis but selection "C" is the *primary* reason for investigation.

28) We selected answer D because:

Geiger-Muller instruments are widely used in survey work and are extremely sensitive to radiation. A discrimination shield is used and when open will admit both gamma and beta emissions. When closed gamma or X-Rays are admitted. The "Cutie pie" is perhaps one of the most widely used instruments available for radiological survey work. They are intended to measure only X-ray and gamma radiation, although some have thin "end-windows" which also allow beta particles measurement. The condenser R-meters are very reliable and accurate instruments for measuring exposures of X and gamma rays. Because of the condenser R-meters great precision, it is frequently used as a secondary standard, but rarely outside of the lab. There is no known device called a "Scatter Absorber".

29) We selected answer B because:

Gases and vapors are most often measured in ppm by volume.

30) We selected answer D because:

A forktruck should never be operated with an overload. This condition removes weight from the steering wheels, which affects the control of the machine. Never add counterweight because it can seriously overload the forks, tires, axles, chains etc.

31)   We selected answer D because:

OSHA requires 19.5% oxygen for all surface work. The scale below describes some problems associated with oxygen-deficient atmospheres.

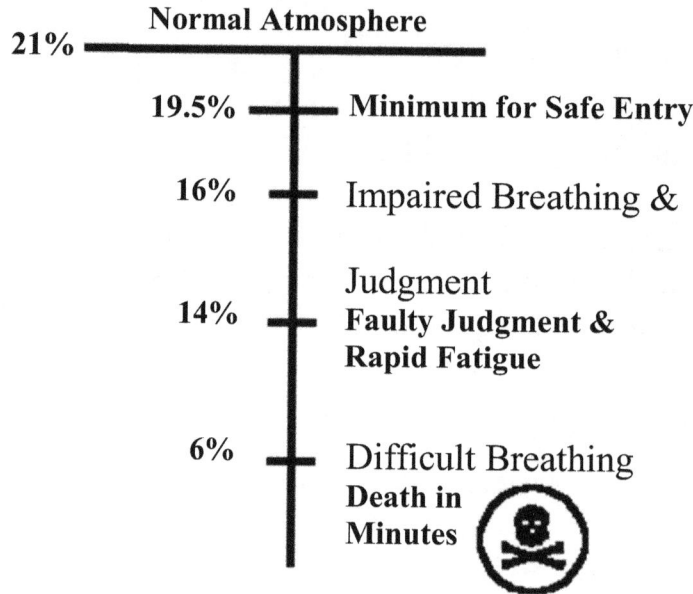

Normal Atmosphere

21% —

19.5% — **Minimum for Safe Entry**

16% — Impaired Breathing &

Judgment
14% — **Faulty Judgment & Rapid Fatigue**

6% — Difficult Breathing
Death in Minutes

32)   We selected answer B because:

Vertical groupings are families and horizontal groupings are periods.

33)   We selected answer B because:

The Atomic number of a substance refers to the total number of protons in the nucleus.

34)   We selected answer D because:

Flammable and combustible liquids are subdivided into classes as shown below (taken from NFPA 30 and 321, *Basic Classification of Flammable and Combustible Liquids*).

FLAMMABLE		
CLASS	Boiling Point	Flash Point
I		below 100 F
IA	below 100 F	below 73 F
IB	at or above 100 F	below 73 F
IC		at or above 73 F and below 100 F
COMBUSTIBLE		

II		at or above 100 F and below 140 F
III		at or above 140 F
IIIA		at or above 140 F and below 200 F
IIIB		at or above 200 F

Note: When a combustible liquid is heated for use to within 30°F of its flashpoint, it must be classified and handled in accordance with the next lowest class of liquid.

35) We selected answer D because:

Sound pressure levels are usually expressed in decibels, however measurement of a "level" is used because the pressure measured is at a level above a given pressure reference. For sound measurements in air the reference is newtons per square meter (N/m^2), dynes per square centimeter (d/cm^2), or microbars. A microbar equals one dyne per square centimeter.

36) We selected answer C because:

If a tagout system is used it must provide full employee protection. This means that the employer must demonstrate that the tagout system will provide a level of safety equivalent to that obtained by using a lockout program. Generally this means the removal of an actuating device eg: the handle on a valve, the removal of a fuse or circuit switch etc.

37) We selected answer B because:

When setting up a straight ladder the base should be one-fourth the ladder length from the vertical plane of the top support.

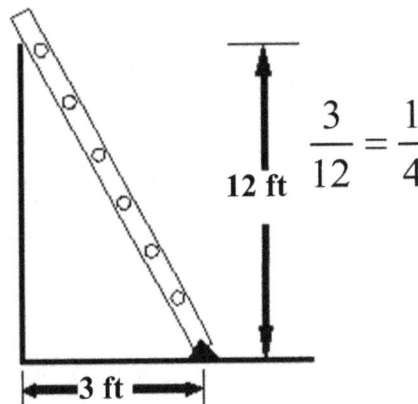

$$\frac{3}{12} = \frac{1}{4}$$

12 ft

3 ft

38) We selected answer C because:

There are two objectives to after training testing. First, to see if the student has gained skill or knowledge in the subject area. Second, to assist the developer and instructor in evaluating the effectiveness of instruction. For example, if a significant percentage of the students in an average class cannot perform up to the specifications outlined in the lesson plans, then the instruction is simply not working. The problem could be the atmosphere, the instructional method, instruction techniques, the instructor, training material, etc. In any event, changes are in order. Effective training is a complex task, in which evaluation of the instruction is often overlooked. One thing that cannot be corrected by training is "poor worker attitude". This is often a complaint against the training staff is that the attitude hasn't changed, but generally that is the responsibility of the supervisor.

39) We selected answer A because:

The molecular weight of dry air is about 30.

40) We selected answer B because:

A combination of non-vented goggles and a face shield provides the *best* protection from the damaging effects of sulfuric acid (H_2SO_4).

41) We selected answer C because:

Specific gravity is the ratio of the weight of one volume of a substance to that of a equal volume of water. Therefore, if a liquid has a specific gravity of 1.2 it is 1.2 times heavier than water.

42) We selected answer B because:

Double insulated equipment does not require a grounding conductor because of the extra protection provided by the additional insulation.

43) We selected answer C because:

Sunlight is the major source of ultraviolet radiation among the sources listed.

44) We selected answer B because:

TLV-STEL (*Threshold Limit Value - Short-Term Exposure Limit*) is the concentration to which workers can be exposed continuously for a short period of time without suffering from:

- Irritation
- Chronic or irreversible tissue damage
- Narcosis of sufficient degree to increase the likelihood of accidental injury, impair self-rescue or materially reduce work efficiency

The STEL is defined as a 15-minute TWA exposure, which should not be exceeded at any time during a work day even if the 8-hour TWA is within the TLV-TWA. Exposures above the TLV-TWA up to the STEL should generally be no longer than 15 minutes for no more than four times per shift. With at least one hour between excursions.

45) We selected answer B because:

Exposed detectors should be examined in bright sunlight or with incandescent lighting. Mercury vapor lighting sometimes makes it difficult to observe color change. Fluorescent lighting should also be avoided because they do not provide a good match for some colors.

46) We selected answer C because:

Specific gravity (sp. gr.) is the ratio of the weight of a certain volume of a liquid or a solid as compared to the weight of an equal volume of water.

47) We selected answer A because:

Although all of the other selections are very important in ensuring an accurate and dependable sampling, placement of the tube in the breathing zone is a primary consideration.

48) We selected answer B because:

Carbon monoxide has about 250 times the affinity of oxygen for the hemoglobin and thus greatly reduces transportation of oxygen.

49) We selected answer D because:

Although all the other answers are factors when using colorimetric sampling devices, interferences by other contaminants is by far the largest single error factor when using these samplers.

50) We selected answer B because:

Grab samples provide instantaneous samples of an atmosphere. Grab sampling is the collection of a sample over a short period of time in an attempt to capture a snapshot of conditions. There are many variables to the art of sampling and grab sampling is a useful tool, however it is generally recognized that long term sampling provides a more in-depth evaluation of the workplace.

51) We selected answer B because:

Moving parts 7 feet or less from the floor must be provided with guarding to prevent inadvertent contact by individuals working in the area.

52) We selected answer B because:

The purpose of local exhaust ventilation is to remove the air contaminants at the source not to dilute them.

53) We selected answer C because:

Safety cans are required to be constructed of fire resistive materials, contain a flame arrestor and a self-closing cover, and be sized to prevent tipping. A fusible link that melts at a pre-determined temperature is not required.

54) We selected answer C because:

OSHA requires 19.5% oxygen for all surface work. The scale below describes some problems associated with oxygen-deficient atmospheres.

55) We selected answer A because:

The employer has the right to refuse entry to an OSHA Compliance Officer or to limit the scope of that inspection as a refusal of entry. However, assuming that the employer does not choose to restrict the OSHA Compliance Officer, the route, timing and scope of inspection is largely up to the inspector. Inspections are either comprehensive or partial. Comprehensive inspections would of course include virtually everything, that is, a wall-to-wall inspection. Partial inspections are limited to certain potentially hazardous areas, operations, conditions or practices at the site. These partial inspections can be expanded based on information gathered by the OSHA Compliance Officer during the inspection process.

56) We selected answer A because:

OSHA provides the following instruction to the OSHA Compliance Safety & Health Officers in the Field Inspection Reference Manual. "At the beginning of the inspection the CSHO shall locate the owner representative, operator or agent in charge at the workplace and present credentials. On construction sites this will most often be the representative of the general contractor. When neither the person in charge nor a management official is present, contact may be made with the employer to request the presence of the owner, operator or management official. The inspection shall not be delayed unreasonably to await the arrival of the employer representative. This delay should normally not exceed one hour. If the person in charge at the workplace cannot be determined, record the extent of the inquiry in the case file and proceed with the physical inspection."

57) We selected answer C because:

OSHA provides the following instruction to the OSHA Compliance Safety & Health Officers in the Field Inspection Reference Manual. "OSHA encourages employers and employees to meet together in the spirit of open communication. The CSHO shall conduct a joint opening conference with employer and employee representatives unless either party objects. If there is objection to a joint conference, the CSHO shall conduct separate conferences with employer and employee representatives."

58) We selected answer B because:

Selection "B" is not correct, the CSHO has no authority to order the closing of an operation or to direct employees to leave the area of imminent danger or the workplace. Selection "A" is true, the CSHO can provide guidance to the employer in developing acceptable abatement methods or provide guidance on seeking appropriate professional assistance. Selection "C" is also correct, if the CSHO does not have all pertinent information at the time of the first closing conference, a second closing conference may be held by telephone. Selection "D" is true.

Although an inspection may be conducted regardless of the existence of a labor dispute involving work stoppage, strikes or picketing, generally a programmed inspection will be deferred until a less troublesome time. The opposite is true of unprogrammed inspections (complaints, fatalities, etc.), which are usually performed even with active labor disputes ongoing.

59) We selected answer B because:

In determining if a hazard is serious or not the question was "Whether the **employer knew**, or with the exercise of reasonable diligence, could have known of the presence of the hazardous condition."

60) We selected answer A because:

Explosion proof equipment is designed to prevent explosions occurring inside the equipment from propagating to the external environment. SEE NFPA 70 ART.500

61) We selected answer C because:

The following information has been extracted and paraphrased from 29 CFR 1926.59. The Hazard Communication Program on multi-employer worksites where the employers produce, use, or store hazardous chemicals in such a way that other employers may be exposed shall develop a program that includes the following:

- The methods the employer will use to provide the other employers with a copy of the MSDS, or make it available at a central location on the worksite.
- The methods the employer will use to inform the other employers of any precautionary measures that need to be taken to protect employees during the workplace's normal operating conditions and in foreseeable emergencies.
- The methods the employer will use to inform the other employers of the labeling system used in the workplace.

62) We selected answer D because:

Labels are required on all of the items listed in the question except the fuel tank on the pickup truck, which is exempt. **1910.1200(f)(5)** Except as provided in paragraphs (f)(6) and (f)(7) of this section, the employer shall ensure that each container of hazardous chemicals in the workplace is labeled, tagged or marked with the following information: identity of the hazardous chemical(s) contained therein; and, appropriate hazard warnings, or alternatively, words, pictures, symbols, or combination thereof, which provide at least general information regarding the hazards of the chemicals, and which, in conjunction with the other information immediately available to employees under the hazard communication program, will provide employees with the specific information regarding the physical and health hazards of the hazardous chemical.

63) We selected answer D because:

To ensure maximum strength has developed in any welded surface, the load transfer from the jacks/lifting units to the building columns, during lift-slab operations, cannot take place until welds on the column shear plates or weld blocks are cooled to air temperature.

64) We selected answer C because:

There are many locations where GFCI are required. However, they are not required in all industrial applications. Additionally, they generally do not function properly when protecting circuits that are extremely long (250 ft. as a rule) because of the capacitive leakage to ground in these circuits. The use of a GFCI is very desirable when using electrical equipment outdoors especially if it is wet, but they are required by Article 680 of the National Electrical Code in and around swimming pools. A few locations where GFCI protection is required include:

- On outdoor receptacles in dwellings where there is grade level access.
- On bathroom receptacles in dwellings.
- On receptacles in dwelling garages (unless circuit includes clothes washers, freezers, garage-door openers etc.
- In kitchens within 6 feet of sinks or grounded metal case appliances.
- On construction sites.
- In and around swimming pools, spas etc.

Remember, the GFCI will not prevent shock, it will render them relatively harmless if installed properly. It will not protect from direct line-to-line contact.

65)   We selected answer B because:

Double or Triple insulated tools do not require equipment grounding due to the extra protection provided by the insulation. Selection "A" is not true, tools that are double or triple insulated do not have to be grounded. Key word here is "ALL". Selection "C" is not true, power operated tools could be used outdoors if the site had an assured grounding program. Selection "D" is not true, GFCIs are not required on construction sites, the alternative is an assured grounding program.

66)   We selected answer B because:

The ear is most susceptible to noise in the range of 1000-4000 Hz.

67)   We selected answer C because:

Hydrocarbons are compounds that contain atoms of carbon and hydrogen only. They are broadly classified into two types, that is; aliphatic and aromatic. *Aliphatic hydrocarbons* are subdivided into saturated and unsaturated compounds and include the alkanes: methane, ethane, propane and butane. *Aromatic hydrocarbons* are derivative of the parent compound benzene. *Ethers* are members of a class of organic compound in which an oxygen atom has bridged between two hydrocarbon groups. Aliphatic ethers are highly volatile and extremely flammable. Hydrocarbons that have been partially halogenated burn, but generally with much less ease than their nonhalogenated analogs. The fully *halogenated* derivatives such as carbon tetrachloride are non-combustible.

68)   We selected answer D because:

The two most common shielded gas welding processes are MIG (Metallic Inert Gas Welding) & TIG (Tungsten Inert Gas). The process is used on Aluminum with a shielding gas of argon or helium. Carbon dioxide would be used as a shield if the process was to be used on steel.

69)   We selected answer C because:

Open frame safety glasses would offer little protection against the toxic effects of a high concentration of acid.

70) We selected answer B because:

Spray paint booths are normally explosive and hazardous when in operation and require Class 1, Division 1 electrical equipment in accordance with ART. 500 of the National Electrical Code. The following table illustrates the classes and divisions of the NEC.

CLASS	DIVISION 1	DIVISION 2
I Gases, Vapors and Liquids (ART. 501)	Normally explosive and hazardous	Not normally present in an explosive concentration (but may accidentally exist)
II Dusts (ART. 502)	Ignitable quantities of dust normally is or may be in suspension or conductive dust may be present	Dust not normally suspended in an ignitable concentration (but may accidentally exist). Dust layers are present
III Fibers and Flyings (ART. 503)	Textiles, woodworking etc. (easily ignitable but not likely to be explosive)	Stored or handled in storage (exclusive of manufacturing)

71) We selected answer B because:

The use of a gas mask is permissible in a IDLH atmosphere due to the presence of a toxic contaminant for escape only.

72) We selected answer D because:

Zero Mechanical State (ZMS) is a common term used in ANSI, OSHA, and other well recognized safety literature and means that all energy sources have been depleted. The system has no residual energy left.

73) We selected answer D because:

When seat belts are required on a vehicle, they must be worn. **1926.602(a)(2)(i)**: Seat belts shall be provided on all equipment covered by this section and shall meet the requirements of the Society of Automotive Engineers, J386-1969, Seat Belts for Construction Equipment. Seat belts for agricultural and light industrial tractors shall meet the seat belt requirements of Society of Automotive Engineers J333a-1970, Operator Protection for Agricultural and Light Industrial Tractors.

1926.602(a)(2)(ii): Seat belts need not be provided for equipment which is designed only for standup operation.

1926.602(a)(2)(iii): Seat belts need not be provided for equipment which does not have roll-over protective structure (ROPS) or adequate canopy protection.

1926.1000(a)(1): This section applies to the following types of material handling equipment: To all rubber-tired, self-propelled scrapers, rubber-tired front-end loaders, rubber-tired dozers, wheel-type agricultural and industrial tractors, crawler tractors, crawler-type loaders, and motor graders, with or without attachments, that are used in construction work. This requirement does not apply to sideboom pipe laying tractors.

1926.1000(b): Equipment manufactured on or after September 1, 1972. Material handling machinery described in paragraph (a) of this section and manufactured on or after September 1, 1972, shall be equipped with rollover protective structures which meet the minimum performance standards prescribed in 1926.1001 and 1926.1002, as applicable.

74) We selected answer C because:

"Contract employer responsibilities."

1926.64(h)(3)(i): The contract employer shall assure that each contract employee is trained in the work practices necessary to safely perform his/her job.

1926.64(h)(3)(ii): The contract employer shall assure that each contract employee is instructed in the known potential fire, explosion, or toxic release hazards related to his/her job and the process, and the applicable provisions of the emergency action plan.

1926.64(h)(3)(iii): The contract employer shall document that each contract employee has received and understood the training required by this paragraph. The contract employer shall prepare a record which contains the identity of the contract employee, the date of training, and the means used to verify that the employee understood the training.

1926.64(h)(3)(iv): The contract employer shall assure that each contract employee follows the safety rules of the facility including the safe work practices required by paragraph (f)(4) of this section.

1926.64(h)(3)(v): The contract employer shall advise the employer of any unique hazards presented by the contract employer's work, or of any hazards found by the contract employer's work.

75) We selected answer A because:

The Ames Test is a very popular quick screening test in use today. The Ames Test or Ames assay is named after its chief developer, Dr. Bruce Ames a biochemist at the University of California at Berkeley. The test uses various strains of Salmonella bacteria to screen suspect chemicals. The test does not measure carcinogenicity directly. It does however measure mutagenicity of a chemical. It is a widely accepted fact that almost all known mutagens are eventually found to be carcinogens. Remember, the test does not measure carcinogenicity directly, but rather the potential for carcinogenicity.

76) We selected answer C because:

1926.760(a)(1)
Except as provided by paragraph (a)(3) of this section, each employee engaged in a steel erection activity who is on a walking/working surface with an unprotected side or edge more than 15 feet (4.6 m) above a lower level shall be protected from fall hazards by guardrail systems, safety net systems, personal fall arrest systems, positioning device systems or fall restraint systems.

1926.760(a)(2)
Perimeter safety cables. On multi-story structures, perimeter safety cables shall be installed at the final interior and exterior perimeters of the floors as soon as the metal decking has been installed.

1926.760(a)(3)
Connectors and employees working in controlled decking zones shall be protected from fall hazards as provided in paragraphs (b) and (c) of this section, respectively.

77) We selected answer B because:

The recommended use of the bar chart is to illustrate comparisons of volume over time

78) We selected answer A because:

Selection "A" is not true. The presence of a combustible mixture causes catalytic combustion on the surface of the hot wire causing an increase in resistance that is converted into a meter movement. The other characteristics of the combustible gas analyzer and the wheatstone bridge circuit are true. A combustible gas monitor is an appropriate instrument when checking concentrations of explosive gases.

79) We selected answer D because:

Article 500 of the NEC deals with classifications of hazardous locations. A hazardous location is defined by the NEC as one in which flammable gases or vapors, flammable liquids, combustible dusts or ignitable flyings or fibers are present in sufficient quantities to require the use of very restrictive wiring and equipment procedures.

80)   We selected answer D because:

The SDS is designed to provide in a concise manner the identification information of a potentially harmful substance together with its hazardous ingredients, physical and chemical characteristics, fire and explosion hazard data, reactivity data, health hazard data, precaution for safe handling/use and control measures. The SDS if the first place you should look for any of the hazardous information. The specific part number of the manufacturer is not required.

81)   We selected answer B because:

All are recommended except notifying the insurance company. Photos are extremely helpful in determining the area of fire origination, the fire suppression system should be checked for proper or improper operation and the fire personnel actions taken need to be documented.

82)   We selected answer A because:

The ABCs of CPR, which stands for airway, breathing and circulation, will aid you in determining what care the victim needs. Determine if the victim's airway is open. Then look, listen and feel for breathing and check for signs of circulation.

83)   We selected answer C because:

According to 40CFR264 –

Sec. 264.37 Arrangements with local authorities.

 The owner or operator must attempt to make the following arrangements, as appropriate for the type of waste handled at his facility and the potential need for the services of these organizations:

  Arrangements to familiarize police, fire departments, and emergency response teams with the layout of the facility, properties of hazardous waste handled at the facility and associated hazards, places where facility personnel would normally be working, entrances to and roads inside the facility, and possible evacuation routes;

No time or distance constraints listed.

Sec. 264.15 General inspection requirements.

> The owner or operator must inspect his facility for malfunctions and deterioration, operator errors, and discharges which may be causing--or may lead to--(1) release of hazardous waste constituents to the environment or (2) a threat to human health. The owner or operator must conduct these inspections often enough to identify problems in time to correct them before they harm human health or the environment.

(b)(1) The owner or operator must develop and follow a written schedule for inspecting monitoring equipment, safety and emergency equipment, security devices, and operating and structural equipment (such as dikes and sump pumps) that are important to preventing, detecting, or responding to environmental or human health hazards.

Sec. 264.52 Content of contingency plan.

> The contingency plan must describe the actions facility personnel must take to comply with Secs. 264.51 and 264.56 in response to fires, explosions, or any unplanned sudden or non-sudden release of hazardous waste or hazardous waste constituents to air, soil, or surface water at the facility.

Sec. 264.13 General waste analysis. (a)(1) Before an owner or operator treats, stores, or disposes of any hazardous wastes, or nonhazardous wastes if applicable under Sec. 264.113(d), he must obtain a detailed chemical and physical analysis of a representative sample of the wastes. At a minimum, the analysis must contain all the information which must be known to treat, store, or dispose of the waste in accordance with this part and part 268 of this chapter.

(b) The owner or operator must develop and follow a written waste analysis plan which describes the procedures which he will carry out to comply with paragraph (a) of this section. He must keep this plan at the facility.

84)   We selected answer B because:

According to OSHA at 1926.152 no more than 25 gallons of flammable or combustible liquids can be stored inside without being in an approved storage cabinet or in a room specifically designed for the storage of flammables/combustibles. The quantity is incorrect in selection "A". Selection "C" incorrectly provides storage in stairwells, which is expressly prohibited. Selection "D" is both unrealistic and incorrect.

85)   We selected answer D because:

For employees who have experienced a significant threshold shift, hearing protector attenuation must be sufficient to reduce employee exposure to a TWA of 85 dB according to OSHA 1910.95 or 1926.52.

86)   We selected answer D because:

Of the equipment listed only the ground impedance tester would indicate the amount of resistance presented to current flow by the equipment ground. All of the other devices would provide an indication of continuity not amount of resistance. An additional piece of equipment that could be used to indicate the amount of resistance would have been the standard volt-ohm meter. However, the difference between the volt-ohm-meter and the ground impedance meter is significant. Impedance checking devices provide information about both high and low current ground faults, whereas the standard volt-ohm-meter would only tell us about protection from low current faults. OSHA at 1910.404 requires two tests. One is a continuity test to ensure that the equipment grounding conductor is electrically continuous. It is performed on all cord sets, receptacles, etc., which are not part of the permanent wiring of the structure. The test may be performed, according to OSHA, using a simple continuity tester such as a lamp and battery, a bell and battery, an ohmmeter, or a receptacle tester. The other test required by OSHA is a polarity check on receptacles and plugs to make sure that the equipment grounding conductor is connected to the correct terminal. The same simple equipment used for the continuity test can be used for this test.

87)   We selected answer B because:

Standard Threshold Shift (STS) is an indicator of hearing loss that may be revealed by an annual audiogram of an employee. As defined in 29 CFR 1910.95, a standard threshold shift is "a change in hearing threshold relative to the baseline audiogram of an average of 10 dB or more at 2,000, 3,000, and 4,000 Hz in either ear." A Hz is one cycle per second.

88)   We selected answer C because:

1910.134(e)(2)(i) The employer shall identify a physician or other licensed health care professional (PLHCP) to perform medical evaluations using a medical questionnaire or an initial medical examination that obtains the same information as the medical questionnaire.

89)   We selected answer D because:

The general agreement within the safety and health community concerning placement of a sound recording instrument microphone is the closer to the workers ear the better. However, the agreed upon definition of hearing zone is a sphere with a two foot diameter surrounding the head. Selection "C" is the preferred definition of Breathing Zone.

90) We selected answer A because:

The Ground-Fault Circuit Interrupter is a fast-action device, which senses a small current leakage to ground and, in a fraction of a second, shuts off the electricity and *interrupts* the faulty flow to ground. Placed between the electrical service and the tool or appliance it serves, the GFCI continually matches the amount of current going to and from the tool along the normal path of the circuit conductors. Whenever the amount *going* differs from the amount *returning* by a set trip level the GFCI interrupts the electric power within 1/40th of a second. This difference in current is called leakage current to ground and the path it takes to ground could be through a person - in which case, the rapid response of the GFCI is fast enough to prevent electrocution. This protection provided by the GFCI is independent of the condition of the equipment grounding conductor, thus, the GFCI can provide protection even if the equipment grounding conductor becomes inoperative. It will however, not detect line-to-line faults.

91) We selected answer D because:

OSHA at 1910.95 and 1926.52 requires exposure to impulsive or impact noise to be limited to 140 dB peak sound pressure level.

92) We selected answer C because:

Stainless steel welding results in fumes containing nickel and chromium. The electrodes used in this process often contain a large amount of fluorides, which are released into the air in large quantities. According to OSHA at 1910.252, "Brazing and gas welding fluxes containing fluorine compounds shall have a cautionary wording to indicate that they contain fluorine compounds. One such cautionary wording recommended by the American Welding Society for brazing and gas welding fluxes reads as follows

CAUTION CONTAINS FLUORIDES

1) This flux when heated gives off fumes that may irritate eyes, nose and throat.

2) Avoid fumes - use only in well-ventilated spaces.
3) Avoid contact of flux with eyes or skin.
4) Do not take internally.

93) We selected answer D because:

The training objectives must be firmly established before a training program is undertaken.

94) We selected answer D because:

Convert percent to ppm and compare to LEL. From the comparison it is obvious that the concentration is above both the PEL and the IDLH but equal to the LEL.

$$ppm = \% \times 1,000,000$$

$$ppm = 2.5\% \times 1,000,000 = 25,000$$

PELs-OSHA Permissible Exposure Limits are time weighted average (TWA) concentrations that must not be exceeded during any 8-hour work shift of a 40-hour workweek.
IDLHs-By NIOSH definition Immediately dangerous to life or health concentrations represent the maximum concentration from which, in the event of respirator failure, one could escape within 30 minutes without a respirator and without experiencing any escape-impairing (e.g., severe eye irritation) or irreversible health effects.
LEL-UEL-Lower Explosive Limit or Lower Flammable Limit. By NFPA definition lower flammable limit is the minimum concentration of vapor to air below which propagation of a flame will not occur in the presence of an ignition source. The UEL or upper flammable limit is the maximum vapor-to-air concentration above which propagation of flame will not occur. At or below the UEL it can ignite. The area bounded by the LEL and the UEL is called the flammability range.

95) We selected answer A because:

Welders have the potential to be exposed to a variety of health hazards. Among these hazards, is fluoride fumes from welding on stainless steel using rods containing fluoride or with some fluxes such as those used in electroslag and submerged arc welding.

96) We selected answer C because:

Overhead cranes can be equipped with a limit switch system to prevent the over travel of the load block. This attachment often referred to as a anti-two block device prevents the load block from being drawn into the sheeve or drum. In the illustration shown here a switch is attached to the crane boom. The switch is held in the closed position by a weight that slides down the hoisting line. When the load block comes too close to the point sheave the weight is lifted and allows the spring loaded switch to open and disconnect power to the hoist apparatus.

97) We selected answer D because:

According to OSHA at 1926.250(b)(6) "Brick stacks shall not be more than 7 feet in height. When a loose brick stack reaches a height of 4 feet, it shall be tapered back 2 inches in every foot of height above the 4-foot level".

98) We selected answer D because:

The following information was extracted from the Hazard Communication Standard "QUIP" published by OSHA. In response to a request for clarification OSHA stated "The HCS sets performance-oriented employee training requirements at section 1926.59 (h) in order to ensure that employees are provided with information and training about the hazardous chemicals they work with, both at the time of their initial assignment and whenever a new hazard is introduced into their work area. However, ..., there is no requirement that "employee training records" be maintained at each jobsite, in fact, there is no requirement in the HCS to maintain any records of employee training."

99) We selected answer C because:

1926.451(g)(1) – Fall Protection
Each employee on a scaffold more than 10 feet (3.1 m) above a lower level shall be protected from falling to that lower level. Paragraphs (g)(1)(i) through (vii) of this section establish the types of fall protection to be provided to the employees on each type of scaffold. Paragraph (g)(2) of this section addresses fall protection for scaffold erectors and dismantlers.
Note to paragraph (g)(1): The fall protection requirements for employees installing suspension scaffold support systems on floors, roofs, and other elevated surfaces are set forth in subpart M of this part.
Each employee on a boatswains' chair, catenary scaffold, float scaffold, needle beam

scaffold, or ladder jack scaffold shall be protected by a personal fall arrest system;
Each employee on a single-point or two-point adjustable suspension scaffold shall be protected by both a personal fall arrest system and guardrail system;
Each employee on a crawling board (chicken ladder) shall be protected by a personal fall arrest system, a guardrail system (with minimum 200 pound toprail capacity), or by a three-fourth inch (1.9 cm) diameter grabline or equivalent handhold securely fastened beside each crawling board;
Each employee on a self-contained adjustable scaffold shall be protected by a guardrail system (with minimum 200 pound toprail capacity) when the platform is supported by the frame structure, and by both a personal fall arrest system and a guardrail system (with minimum 200 pound toprail capacity) when the platform is supported by ropes;

100)   We selected answer D because:

Bonding is the process of connecting two or more conductive objects together by means of a conductor to minimize the potential electrical difference between them. Grounding is the process of connecting the conductive objective to the ground and is a specific type of bonding. A conductive object may also be grounded by bonding it to another conductive object that is already connected to the ground. *Bonding* minimizes potential differences between conductive objects. *Grounding* minimizes potential differences between conductive objects and the ground. In dealing with flammable liquids, both *Bonding and Grounding* are very important.

Self-Assessment Exam Four Questions

1) Which of the following "Laws of Learning" is characterized by the ability of students to remember the task they learned last?

  A) Law of Frequency.
  B) Law of Recency.
  C) Law of Effect.
  D) Law of Readiness.

2) The Mine Safety and Health Administration (MSHA) requires certain training for each new underground miner. Which of the following **best** describes that training?

  A) Performance based training.
  B) Specification based training.
  C) 180 hours of on-the-job training.
  D) 10 hours of classroom education.

3) An OSHA Compliance Safety and Health Officer is making an inspection and observes several hazardous containers of chemicals without any label. During a short investigation, the Compliance Officer determines that the containers were received without labels. Can the Compliance Officer issue a citation?

  A) Yes, the employer can be cited unless good faith efforts have been made to obtain a proper label.
  B) No, the supplier will be cited.
  C) Yes, both will be cited.
  D) No, labels fall off all the time.

4) An instrument which can be used to read an electrical current in a circuit without tapping the circuit is?

  A) A megger.
  B) Glavometer.
  C) Split core ammeter.
  D) Standard volt-ohm meter.

5) The A-weighted sound level measurement is used as the "standard" scale in occupational noise measurement because:
- A) It weights intermittent and impact noise.
- B) Weighting is related to effects of noise on the ear.
- C) It filters out "white" noise.
- D) It has a built-in dose response curve.

6) The recommended rating of a firewall separating oxygen and fuel gases should be how high?
- A) 3 feet.
- B) 5 feet.
- C) 7 feet.
- D) 9 feet.

7) Ladder jack scaffold platforms shall not exceed a height of ____feet?
- A) 10.
- B) 20.
- C) 25.
- D) 30.

8) The OSHA form 300 must be retained in the workplace for:
- A) 1 year.
- B) 5 years.
- C) 30 years.
- D) 15 years.

9) When doing training for welders on the fire characteristics of liquid hazardous chemicals which of the following would **not** be discussed?
- A) TLV.
- B) Autoignition temperature.
- C) Lower Explosive Limit.
- D) Upper Flammable Limit.

10) You are conducting a training session, which illustrates the principles of Industrial Hygiene sampling techniques, the class is divided into two sessions, personal sampling and general-area sampling. During this training session a student asks the question - What are the two **most common** solid-sorbent tubes used in air sampling? Your response should be:

    A)   Porapak P and Ambersorb.
    B)   Ambersorb and Silica gel.
    C)   Charcoal and Tenax-GC.
    D)   Charcoal and Silica gel.

11) The 3 in the diagram indicates:
    A)   Health.
    B)   Fire.
    C)   Reactivity.
    D)   Storage.

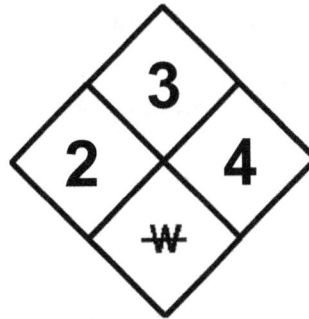

12) Which of the following statements **best** describes the OSHA Hazard Communication Standard (HCS)?

A) The HCS is a standard that applies to every citizen of the United States.
B) The HCS does not apply to construction.
C) The HCS is a specification-based standard.
D) The HCS is a performance standard.

13) The Life Safety Code is:

  A) FM Standard Number 1.
  B) Uniform Building Code Number 1.
  C) An old standard from the 1940s.
  D) NFPA 101.

14) All of the following statements concerning the OSHA Hazard Communication program are false **except?**

  A) Training must be done annually.
  B) SDS requirements apply to free samples.
  C) Labels can be in Spanish if your workforce is over 85% Spanish speaking.
  D) SDS must be kept for 5 years.

15) Which of the following is true concerning the training of personnel who erect and dismantle scaffolding?

  A) Training must be done under the supervision of a certified training instructor.
  B) A competent person must perform the training.
  C) Training is not, and never was required.
  D) Training is a good idea and would ensure safety but is not required by OSHA.

16) During the planning stage of a Construction Health & Safety Training Program, which of the following is the **most important** consideration?
  A) Training Objectives.
  B) Training Methods.
  C) Instructor Qualifications.
  D) Training Program Content.

17) Which of the following is **not** a duty of a Central Safety Committee?
  A) Approve purchase requests for safety equipment.
  B) Review design of new plant equipment.
  C) Investigate extra hazardous conditions.
  D) Guide and direct the safety effort.

18) Your company has hired a new worker who was qualified as a powered truck operator at her previous company. What is the training required to get this person qualified as a power truck operator in your company?

    A) Send to a formal school.
    B) Accept the other company's qualification.
    C) Have the employee attend your company's initial training program.
    D) Ensure the operator has the knowledge and skills required to operate the power trucks, including your company's procedures.

19) The primary purpose for using On-the-Job training is:
    A) It is cost effective.
    B) More than one person can be trained at a time.
    C) Requires the minimum amount of time for total training.
    D) Allows the worker to produce during the training period.

20) A needs assessment does all the following **except?**

    A) Identifies the type of training required.
    B) Identifies the problem or need before designing a solution.
    C) Saves time and money by ensuring that solutions effectively address the problems they are intended to solve.
    D) Identifies factors that will impact the training before its development.

21) Which of the following is the **best indicator** of training effectiveness?

    A) Favorable Student Critiques.
    B) Correct Student Response to Questions.
    C) Increase in effectiveness of Job Performance.
    D) Testing meets expected norms.

22) Verbs or actions words used in learning objectives must be as specific as possible. The behavior must be observable and measurable. Which of the following verbs does **not** meet this criterion?

    A) Understand.
    B) Identify.
    C) Troubleshoot.
    D) Enter data.

23) Employee training records maintained under the provisions of 1910.1030 must be retained for what period of time?

    A) 3 years from the date of training.
    B) Duration of employment plus 3 years.
    C) 5 years from the date of training.
    D) Duration of employment plus 5 years.

24) When required to use PPE, the employee must be training in all the areas **except?**

    A) How to purchase PPE.
    B) When PPE is necessary.
    C) The limitations of the PPE .
    D) How to properly don, doff, adjust, and wear PPE.

25) During a training session on hazardous material labeling, you are referring to the NFPA 704, Identification of Hazards of Materials. During this presentation you should properly identify what color and purpose for the left diamond?

    A) Blue, fire.
    B) Yellow, fire.
    C) Red, fire.
    D) Blue, health.

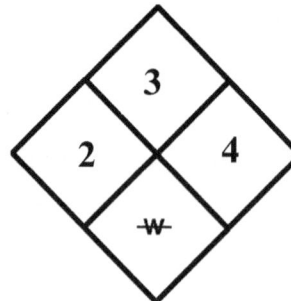

26) Successful adult training can be measured by all of the following **except?**

    A) Demonstrate the application.
    B) Show a tape of a previous experience.
    C) Let the trainee practice the new skill.
    D) Discuss how the new skills can be applied.

27) Which of the following is **not** an expected outcome of group training?

    A) Gain skills.
    B) Share ideas.
    C) Evaluate information.
    D) Become actively involved in the planning and implementation of company policy.

28) Permit required confined spaces requires all of the following training **except?**

    A) Annually.
    B) Before the employee is assigned or there is a change in duty assignments.
    C) Whenever there is a change in permit space operations that introduces a new hazard.
    D) Whenever there are deviations from the company procedures or the employee requires retraining.

29) Which of the following Internet connections will provide you with the **greatest** bandwidth?

    A) ISP.
    B) T-1.
    C) DSL.
    D) Telephone Service.

30) Training on the hazards that cause lung disease would often include "pneumoconiosis", sometimes called dusty lung. What is the pneumoconiosis that is caused by inhalation of iron oxide called?

    A) Anthracosis.
    B) Siderosis.
    C) Silicosis.
    D) Silicosiderosis.

31) Training on Industrial Hygiene sampling practices often includes the use of various detector tubes. Which of the following is the **largest** source of error when using colorimetric sampling devices?
   A) Charcoal packed too tight.
   B) Channeling.
   C) Temperature extremes.
   D) Interference from other contaminants.

32) Which of the following is the **best** statement concerning interchanging colorimetric tubes obtained from various manufacturers?
   A) Interchanging tubes is never permitted.
   B) Interchanging tubes is always permitted.
   C) Interchanging tubes is sometimes permitted.
   D) Interchanging tubes is allowed as long as the pump quantities are the same.

33) Training on hazardous materials often includes definitions. When the vapor pressure of a liquid is greater than the atmospheric pressure, this is known as the:
   A) Flash point (closed cup).
   B) Flash point (open cup)
   C) Boiling point.
   D) Freezing point.

34) Who is in the **best** position to provide effective safety training of industrial work groups?
   A) Supervisors.
   B) Senior Management.
   C) OHSTs.
   D) Training Professionals.

35) Which of the following would **not** be an accurate statement to be included in a training session about the characteristics of colorimetric tubes when doing Industrial Hygiene Sampling?
   A) Tubes are cheap and easy to read.
   B) Tubes are very accurate.
   C) Tubes are affected by contaminates in the air.
   D) Tubes have a long shelf life.

36) ANSI Z16.2 "Method of recording basic facts relating to the nature and occurrence of work injuries" contains an analytical category called accident, that identifies the object, substance, or premises that contained a hazardous condition. This category is called?

    A) Hazard index.
    B) Agency of Accident.
    C) Hazardous Condition.
    D) Accident Classification.

37) During a Industrial Hygiene class demonstrating sampling techniques the following statement is made, "colorimetric tubes are often used in routine measurements in the Safety & Health field". Which of the following explanations **best** describes the wide use of these tubes?

    A) One tube can be used for a large number of samples.
    B) One tube can be used for a large number of contaminates.
    C) Tubes are cheap and easy to read.
    D) Tubes are expensive but provide very precise results.

38) If a personnel platform is attached to a hydraulic crane, then?

    A) It is not authorized.
    B) May only be used on situations authorized by OSHA.
    C) Does not require any special procedures or pretesting.
    D) A trial lift with the unoccupied personnel platform loaded at least to the anticipated lift weight shall be made.

39) Wire rope shall not be used if, in any length of eight diameters, the total number of visible broken wires exceeds ___ percent of the total number of wires, or if the rope shows other signs of excessive wear, corrosion, or defect.

    A) 5.
    B) 7.5.
    C) 10.
    D) 15.

40) Compressed gas cylinders in storage must be separated from other combustible material by a barrier that is non-combustible, has as 30 minute fire rating and is at least ____ feet high?
    A) 3.
    B) 5.
    C) 7.
    D) 10.

41) Any employee engaged in a steel erection activity who is on a walking/working surface with an unprotected side or edge more than ___ feet (4.6 m) above a lower level shall be protected from fall hazards by guardrail systems, safety net systems, personal fall arrest systems, positioning device systems or fall restraint systems.
    A) 6.
    B) 10.
    C) 15.
    D) 20.

42) Which of the following is Public Law 91-596?
    A) Occupational Safety and Health Act.
    B) Federal Coal Mine Health and Safety Act.
    C) Federal Metal and Nonmetallic Mine Safety Act.
    D) Federal Mine Safety and Health Act.

43) Which of the following is the common language of client/server database management?
    A) SQL.
    B) URL.
    C) HTML.
    D) HTTP.

44) You are transiting the production area and spot a safety hazard that presents imminent danger to the workers in the area. Your first action should be to:
    A) Shut down the production line.
    B) Fix the hazard.
    C) Post a lock-out/tag-out sign until the hazard is corrected.
    D) Notify the area supervisor to get the hazard corrected

45) In order to provide a safe work place, the safety professional should:

  A) Always seek an outside opinion before making a decision.
  B) Consult the local ASSE chapter for guidance when needed.
  C) Make decisions on all situations based on their knowledge.
  D) Limit their advice and recommendation to those areas that they have knowledge in.

46) Once you obtained your CHST, you must maintain your currency in the safety and health arena. This is monitored by the BCSP by the Certification Maintenance program. If you fail to meet your required 20 points in five years you must:

  A) Obtain 50 points in the next five-year period.
  B) Complete 20 college credits to be reinstated.
  C) Retake the CHST exam.
  D) Resubmit an application for reevaluation.

47) You are conducting a safety inspection of a manufacturing plant in the southwest. The inspection is designed to fulfill two purposes, one to indoctrinate a new junior safety engineer, and second to uncover non-compliance with federal, state and local directives. During your inspection you observe an employee, without eye protection, working at a bench installing parts. This is not a hazardous operation but it is a posted "eye protection" area. Which of the following is the **best** course of action?

  A) Contact the supervisor and discuss the situation.
  B) Test the junior safety engineer's skills by letting her handle the situation.
  C) Confront the employee and determine "Why" eye protection is not being used.
  D) Note the discrepancy and do not discuss it until the out brief when the CEO and the supervisor are both present.

48) During an OSHA inspection of a multiemployer worksite the OSHA Compliance Safety & Health Officer (CSHO) observes an employee using an obviously substandard tool belt as a fall protection device. Who will the CSHO most likely cite for the unsafe belt?

   A)   The owner.
   B)   The employee.
   C)   The subcontractor.
   D)   The general and the subcontractor.

49) After a training session to introduce a set of employees to a new process, you pass out an evaluation sheet to obtain feedback from the employees on the training session. Which of the following would be an inappropriate question?

   A)   Was the content accurate?
   B)   Did the instructor display enthusiasm?
   C)   Did the instructor maintain your interest?
   D)   Was the presentation organized/easy to follow?

50) The **best** way to deal with minor infractions of work or safety rules?

   A)   Oral reprimand.
   B)   Written reprimand.
   C)   Ignore it.
   D)   Suspension.

51) On a multi-employer worksite, the general contractor has agreed to act as an intermediary for storage of the MSDSs for the entire site. An OSHA inspector found several containers of hazardous chemicals without a label or MSDS in a sub-contractor's trailer. A short investigation by the Compliance Officer revealed that the sub-contractor failed to notify the general that he had the hazardous materials. Who would be cited for this violation?

   A)   Both the general and the sub-contractor.
   B)   The owner.
   C)   The general contractor.
   D)   The sub-contractor.

52) When you measure training program effectiveness, which of the following is the **least valuable?**

   A) Behavior – what behaviors were changed as a result of the training.
   B) Knowledge – what skills were learned and demonstrated.
   C) Reaction – how the students liked the training.
   D) Interaction – how the students interacted and exchanged ideas in class.

53) Under the provisions of the OSHA Hazard Communication Standard, who has the responsibility to determine if a material is hazardous?

   A) All employees have this right.
   B) The manufacturer or importer of the chemical.
   C) The employer is legally obligated to make this determination.
   D) Unionized employees have this right.

54) If CHSTs were petitioning to the state to have only certified individual recognized as safety and health professionals, this would be an example of:

   A) Title Protection.
   B) Professional Registration.
   C) A Title Act.
   D) Professional Competence Standard.

55) Which of the following reflects the **best** use of the management tool, Failure Modes and Effects Analysis (FMEA)?

   A) Survey instrument.
   B) Inspection checklist.
   C) Preventative maintenance indicator.
   D) Alternate for fault tree.

56) Which of the following responsibilities is **not** assigned to the National Institute for Occupational Safety and Health (NIOSH)?

   A) Research and identification of occupational safety/health hazards.
   B) Recommending changes to safety/health regulations.
   C) Training of safety/health personnel.
   D) Enforcement of occupational safety/public health standards within the regulated community.

57) A staff safety engineer is given the authority by the General Manager to stop operations on a construction site whenever he or she observes an imminent danger situation. Which of the following correctly identifies the authority granted by the General Manager?

   A) Staff authority.
   B) Staff to line authority.
   C) Authority of delegation.
   D) Functional authority.

58) "Access to employee exposure and medical records", is applicable to construction operations and requires that workplace monitoring data be maintained by the employer. How long do these records have to be kept?

   A) 30 years.
   B) Duration of employment plus 30 years.
   C) 5 years.
   D) Duration of employment plus 5 years.

59) The CHST certification is sponsored through:

   A) ABIH.
   B) BCSP.
   C) ASSE.
   D) NSC.

60) Which of the following encompasses the term *non-combustible*?

   A) Fire proof.
   B) Fire resistive.
   C) Flame proof.
   D) Fire retardant.

61) Several methods of securing line accountability for safety are widely accepted within the safety community. Which of the following techniques will have long lasting influence on the line manager or supervisor?
   A) Charge accidents to departments.
   B) Put safety in supervisor's appraisal.
   C) Have safety affect supervisor's income.
   D) All of the above.

62) In 1970, Congress passed the Occupational Safety and Health Act (OSHA), which mandated the use of many safety standards by several industries. The OSHA construction safety standards are known as?
   A) CFR 49.
   B) CFR 30.
   C) 29 CFR 1910.
   D) 29 CFR 1926.

63) The OSHA DART is frequently used in industrial safety work. This indicator should be used as:
   A) An absolute rate to compare with other industries.
   B) An indicator of serious injury frequency.
   C) A yardstick after converting to a million man-hours.
   D) An accident severity rate to compare your severity and frequency against other similar industry rates.

64) You have been called on to determine the correct fire suppression agent for a fire involving a combustible metal used in your plant. Which agent would you choose?
   A) Green triangle with an A in the center.
   B) Red square with a B in the center.
   C) Blue circle with a C in the center.
   D) Yellow star with a D in the center.

65)	One of the most important functions of management is to set goals and objectives. Which of the following methods is used as a tool to accomplish this task?

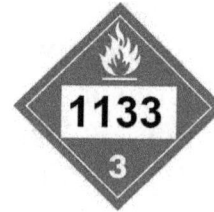

   A)	Performance review.
   B)	MBO system.
   C)	Zero based budgeting.
   D)	None of the above.

66)	What types of ladders are approved for electrical work?

   A)	Metal.
   B)	Only wooden ladders.
   C)	Nonconductive ladders, including wooden.
   D)	Ladders are not approved for electrical work.

67)	What does the number "3" indicate on the Hazardous Material Label?

   A)	Flammable material.
   B)	Adhesive material.
   C)	Hazard class.
   D)	Third label in the series.

68)	All of the following are required steps to perform chain-of-custody on evidence collected during an accident investigation **except?**

   A)	Collect.
   B)	Track.
   C)	Identify.
   D)	Log movement.

69)	Whenever materials are dropped more than ____ feet to any point lying outside the exterior walls of the building, an enclosed chute of wood, or equivalent material, shall be used. For the purpose of this paragraph, an enclosed chute is a slide, closed in on all sides, through which material is moved from a high place to a lower one.

   A)	20.
   B)	30.
   C)	40.
   D)	Not required.

70) Which of the following is **not** a characteristic of local exhaust ventilation, when compared to dilution ventilation:

    A) Is more suitable for highly toxic substances.
    B) Is very good for ventilating point source emissions.
    C) Costs less than dilution ventilation.
    D) Uses less air than dilution ventilation.

71) The minimum amount of electric current passing through the body to produce a fatality is:

    A) 7 amps.
    B) 2 amps.
    C) 500-750 mA.
    D) 70-100 mA.

72) In general, personal protective equipment tends to increase worker efficiency and decrease personnel injury.

    A) True for all industries.
    B) False.
    C) Only true for construction.
    D) Only false for fall protection because it hinders movement.

73) OSHA recommends what level of lighting for general construction area work?

    A) 5 footcandles.
    B) 10 footcandles.
    C) 15 footcandles.
    D) 20 footcandles.

74) Which of the following conditions would cause a safety professional the **most concern?**

    A) Working in a 13 psia atmosphere.
    B) Working in a 120° F atmosphere.
    C) Heat load of 3500 BTU per hour.
    D) Airflow resulting in one air change every five minutes.

75) Which of the following statements is **most correct** concerning electrical Ground Fault Circuit Interrupters (GFCI)?

    A) GFCIs will trip at about 5 milliamps line-to-line fault current.

    B) GFCIs will trip at about 5 milliamps line-to-ground fault current.

    C) GFCIs will protect against line to ground and line to line faults and trip at about 15 amperes.

    D) GFCIs are required on all construction sites .

76) What is the maximum storage temperature for a gas cylinder?

    A) 100° F.

    B) 100° C.

    C) 130° F.

    D) 130° C.

77) The two types of systems used to control the volume of air movements in a ventilation system are:

    A) Blast Gate and Slot Reduction.

    B) Blast Gate and Balance by Design.

    C) Balance by Design and Slot Reduction.

    D) Open-Close Gate and Unbalanced Closure.

78) How often is calibration of sound level meters required?

    A) Monthly.

    B) Quarterly.

    C) Before each survey.

    D) Before and after each survey.

The following tables were extracted from 1926 Subpart P Appendix C and are to be used for the following 3 questions.

Table C-1.1

Timber Trenching Shoring- Minimum Timber Requirements*

Soil Type A P_a = 25 x H + 72 psf (2 ft Surcharge)

Depth of Trench (feet)	Size (actual) and spacing of members**													
	Cross braces							Wales		Uprights				
	Horiz. Spacing (feet)	Width of trench (feet)					Vertical Spacing (feet)	Size (in.)	Vertical Spacing (feet)	Maximum allowable Horizontal spacing				
		Up to 4	Up to 6	Up to 9	Up to 12	Up to 15				Close	4	5	6	8
5 to 10	Up to 6	4 x 4	4 x 4	4 x 6	6 x 6	6 x 6	4	NR	--				2 x 6	
	Up to 8	4 x 4	4 x 4	4 x 6	6 x 6	6 x 6	4	NR	--					2x 6
	Up to 10	4 x 6	4 x 6	4 x 6	6 x 6	6 x 6	4	8 x 8	4			2x 6		
	Up to 12	4 x 6	4 x 6	6 x 6	6 x 6	6 x 6	4	8 x 8	4				2 x 6	
10 to 15	Up to 6	4 x 4	4 x 4	4 x 6	6 x 6	6 x 6	4	NR	--				3 x 8	
	Up to 8	4 x 4	4 x 4	4 x 6	6 x 6	6 x 6	4	8 x 8	4		2x 6			
	Up to 10	4 x 6	4 x 6	6 x 6	6 x 6	6 x 6	4	8x 10	4			2x 6		
	Up to 12	6 x 6	6 x 6	6 x 6	6 x 8	6 x 8	4	10 x 10	4				2x 8	
15 to 20	Up to 6	6 x 6	6 x 6	6 x 6	6 x 8	6 x 8	4	6 x 8	4	3 x 6				
	Up to 8	6 x 6	6 x 6	6 x 6	6 x 8	6 x 8	4	8 x 8	4	3 x 6				
	Up to 10	8 x 8	8 x 8	8 x 8	8 x 8	8x10	4	8 x 10	4	3 x 6				
	Up to 12	8 x 8	8 x 8	8 x 8	8 x 8	8x10	4	10 x 10	4	3 x 6				
Over 20	See Note 1													

Mixed oak or equivalent with a bending strength not less than 850 psi

** Manufactured members of equivalent strength may be substituted for wood.

Table C-1.3
Timber Trenching Shoring- Minimum Timber Requirements*
Soil Type C $P_a = 80 \times H + 72$ psf (2 ft Surcharge)

Depth of Trench (feet)	Size (actual) and spacing of members**										
	Cross braces							Wales		Uprights	
	Horiz. Spacing (feet)	Width of trench (feet)					Vertical Spacing (feet)	Size (in.)	Vertical Spacing (feet)	Maximum allowable Horizontal spacing (feet) See Note 2	
		Up to 4	Up to 6	Up to 9	Up to 12	Up to 15				Close	
5 to 10	Up to 6	6 x 8	6 x 8	6 x 8	8 x 8	8 x 8	5	8x10	5	2 x 6	
	Up to 8	8 x 8	8 x 8	8 x 8	8 x 8	8 x 10	5	10 x 12	5	2 x 6	
	Up to 10	8x10	8x10	8x10	8x10	10 x 10	5	12 x 12	5	2 x 6	
	See Note 1										
10 to 15	Up to 6	8 x 8	8 x 8	8 x 8	8 x 8	8 x 10	5	10 x 12	5	2 x 6	
	Up to 8	8x10	8x10	8x10	8x10	10 x 10	5	12 x 12	5	2 x 6	
	See Note 1										
	See Note 1										
15 to 20	Up to 6	8x10	8x10	8x10	8x10	10 x 10	5	12 x 12	5	3 x 6	
	See Note 1										
	See Note 1										
	See Note 1										
Over 20	See Note 1										

Mixed oak or equivalent with a bending strength not less than 850 psi.
Mixed oak or equivalent with a bending strength not less than 850 psi
** Manufactured members of equivalent strength may be substituted for wood.

79) You need to select shoring material for a trench in Type C soil that is 13 feet deep and 5 feet wide. The cross braces will be spaced at 6 feet horizontally and 5 feet vertically, what size of timber is required?

    A)   4 x 4.
    B)   8 x 8.
    C)   8 x 10.
    D)   10 x 10.

80) You need to select shoring material for a trench in Type A soil that is 17 feet deep and 8 feet wide. The cross braces will be spaced at 10 feet horizontally and 4 feet vertically, what size of timber is required?

    A)   4 x 4.
    B)   6 x 6.
    C)   8 x 8.
    D)   8 x 10.

81) You need to select shoring material for a trench in Type C soil that is 25 feet deep and 5 feet wide. The cross braces will be spaced at 4 feet horizontally and 5 feet vertically, what size of timber is required?

    A)   8 x 10.
    B)   10 x 10.
    C)   Design by a registered CSP.
    D)   Design by a registered professional engineer.

82) During Health and Safety communications with workers, the main objective is to?

    A)   Teach workers to understand what is begin said.
    B)   Provide a vehicle for suggestions.
    C)   Teach workers to write and read well.
    D)   Provide a safety message that will be understood and accepted by the workers.

83) Under provisions of the OSHAct, employers can be cited for repeated violations if that employer has been cited previously for a substantially similar condition. This sounds simple enough, however it becomes complicated especially if an employer has multiple worksites. Is a citation a repeat if it happens in a different state a year later? Which of the following is the **most correct** concerning the repeat citation policy of OSHA?

   A) Violations will be considered repeat if they occur within one year of each other.
   B) Violations will be considered repeat if they occur within 6 months of each other.
   C) Violations will be considered repeat if they occur within five years of each other.
   D) Violations will be considered repeat if they occur within three years of each other.

84) If an employer who was required by OSHA to maintain injury and illness records sells the company, does the new owner need to maintain the log and other injury records from the old owner?

   A) No, each owner is responsible for their own records.
   B) No, but if OSHA inspects they may want to see the records from the old owner.
   C) Yes, the new owner must get the records from the old owner and keep them the appropriate time period.
   D) Yes, but the old owner is entirely responsible for the records and must do any updating or maintenance required until the end of the retention period.

85) A carpenter was injured on the job when he ran a splinter into his arm. He went to see the on-site Registered Nurse (RN) who removed the splinter and cleaned the puncture. The RN said he would not need additional treatment, however she requested he return the next day for observation. Which of the following is the **best** OSHA classification for the incident?

   A) First-aid injury.
   B) Recordable lost time injury.
   C) Medical treatment, greater than first-aid.
   D) Not recordable less than first aid.

86) According to the OSHA Hazard Communication Standard, all of the following are valid requirements and would require employers to provide employees training on the hazardous chemicals in the workplace, **except?**

    A) Restocking of chemicals.
    B) New chemical hazard in the work environment.
    C) Change in job assignment with new chemicals.
    D) Initial assignment.

87) Hazard control can be accomplished in a variety of ways. Common methods of hazard control include: using personal protective equipment, reducing exposure, designing out the hazard and eliminating the hazard by substitution or automation. What is the order of precedence of these hazard control methods from highest to lowest?

    A) Using personal protective equipment, designing out the hazard, and eliminating the hazard by substitution or automation, reducing exposure.
    B) Eliminating the hazard by substitution or automation, designing out the hazard, reducing exposure, and using personal protective equipment.
    C) Designing out the hazard, eliminating the hazard by substitution or automation, reducing exposure, and using personal protective equipment.
    D) Designing out the hazard, eliminating the hazard by substitution or automation, using personal protective equipment, and reducing exposure.

88) Which of the following factors does **not** affect the load capacity of a mobile crane?
    A) Boom length.
    B) Boom angle.
    C) Extension of outriggers.
    D) Installation of anti-two-blocking device.

89) Which is a direct cause:
    A) Human error.
    B) SOP was not followed.
    C) Equipment malfunction caused injury.
    D) Ignoring a safety rule.

90) Training mandated by the Hazard Communication Standard is accomplished to allow employees to become familiar with the hazards of chemicals in the workplace and protective measures. Which of the following statements is the **most correct** concerning Hazcom training done by a commercial training company?

    A) OSHA will cite both the employer and the training company for any training deficiencies.

    B) OSHA will cite the training company only if it has been licensed and approved by OSHA.

    C) OSHA will cite the commercial training company for any training deficiencies.

    D) OSHA will cite the employer for any training deficiencies.

91) The fire tetrahedron states that combustion requires an oxidizer, fuel, heat and which of the following?

    A) Confinement.

    B) Surface area.

    C) Chain reaction.

    D) Deflagration.

92) Which of the following professionals is dedicated to the art and science of anticipation, recognition, evaluation and control of those environmental factors in the workplace that may cause sickness, impaired health and well-being?

    A) Industrial Hygienist.

    B) Industrial Toxicologist.

    C) Health Physicist.

    D) Medical Pathologist.

93) What should the safety professional ensure was considered before retraining the employees as a recommendation for corrective action?

    A) That requiring employees 10 complete a written checklist bad been considered.

    B) That requiring employees to don personal protective equipment had been considered.

    C) That one or more effective engineering controls had been considered.

    D) That one or more effective administrative controls had been considered.

94) Which of the following is the **most essential** when conducting a successful hazard and operability study?
- A) Multiple union and management representatives familiar with safety procedures.
- B) A study leader familiar with the process being studied.
- C) A knowledgeable process safety engineer familiar with process safety regulations.
- D) Multiple subject matter experts knowledgeable about the process being studied.

95) As a new safety manager, you have been ask to develop an incident data collection system. What is the **most important** first step in this process?
- A) Identify existing data sources and codify the data.
- B) Establish incident reporting procedures.
- C) Define the subsequent use of the data.
- D) Define investigation team parameters.

96) Which device is **best** for measuring an employee's accumulated radiation dose?
- A) Portacount.
- B) Currie counter.
- C) Pocket dosimeter.
- D) Geiger counter.

97) In addition to the metal fumes, metal oxides, and the products of combustion from vaporized paints and coatings from the welded items, what hazardous gas is produced during electric arc welding?
- A) Hydrogen peroxide.
- B) Diacetyl.
- C) Ozone.
- D) Diethylamine.

98) Because of high eye and foot injury rates, management at a union labor manufacturing plant must take action. Which action should a safety professional perform first?

    A) Survey the facilities and operations to determine probable causes of the injuries.

    B) Initiate a personal protective equipment program that will include provision of both safety glasses with side shields and hard-toed shoes.

    C) Schedule a meeting with the head of the local union to review the injury problems.

    D) Charter a facility-wide safety committee.

99) Which is an example of a well-constructed training objective?

    A) Students will understand the safety policy.

    B) General industry training standards.

    C) Each student can demonstrate the proper Electrical Procedures.

    D) Supervisors will be motivated deliver safety training.

100) Which of the following is **not** considered a basic principle of loss control?

    A) "An unsafe act, an unsafe condition, and an accident are all symptoms of something wrong in the management system."

    B) We can predict that certain sets of circumstances will produce severe injuries. These circumstances can be identified and controlled."

    C) "The key to effective line safety performance is management procedures that fix accountability."

    D) "Safety must be managed as a special company function - set apart from the normal planning process to ensure management's commitment to safety is clearly visible among employees."

Self-Assessment Exam Four Answers

1) We selected answer B because:

The "Laws of Learning" are as follows:

Law of Recency: People tend to recall and use that which they learned last or most recently. It is easier to remember a subject after a recent seminar, or how to solve a complex technical problem on the job, than to recall a simple trigonometry problem from high school.

Law of Frequency: The more often a mental connection is made, the stronger it becomes. Repetition is helpful in skill and attitude development and habit formation.

Law of Effect: People like to do things which bring pleasure and enjoyment. They learn easily and quickly those things that are pleasant experiences and they remember these things longer.

Law of Readiness: People must be in a receptive frame of mind if the learning is to be effective... that is, ready to see the value of learning a particular thing as a benefit to them. We all learn more easily if we see the value and desire to learn.

Law of Disuse: When knowledge or a skill is not used it becomes *fuzzy* or *rusty* and is more difficult to recall or use because it isn't used. Knowledge is the first to suffer from disuse, skill may become rusty, but often are quickly relearned with a little practice.

Law of Primacy: People learn things that are important to them and have special meaning to their lives. These are primary to them and will often ease the difficulty in learning complex skills or knowledge.

Law of Intensity: The more involved we become in learning, the more we learn and the better we learn. Active learning from reading, and performing a skill are superior to passive learning from watching a movie. Learning is an individual effort and the more we involve individual participation, the stronger the experience.

2) We selected answer B because:

Throughout the history of The Mine Safety and Health Administration (MSHA) the organization has stressed the importance of training for miners. The training is expressly prescribed, "Every new underground miner shall receive no less than 40 hours of prescribed training". MSHA then lists the prescribed training complete with format. This is in contrast to the performance based training required by recent legislation (e.g.: the OSHA Hazard Communication Standard).

3) We selected answer A because:

If labels or MSDSs are missing or have not been received for a hazardous chemical, the employer will be cited unless a good faith effort has been made to obtain the information. Good faith efforts may include a documented phone call or letter to the supplier or you may call OSHA and request help in securing the label or MSDS.

4) We selected answer C because:

A split core ammeter has fingers that enclose the conductor under test without opening or tapping the circuit. This is much safer than other methods.

5) We selected answer B because:

The A-weighing most closely weights the sound to the injurious effects of the noise on the ear.

6) We selected answer B because:

The OSHA at 1910.252 requires the separation of oxygen and fuel gas cylinders by 20 feet or a one half hour wall at least 5 feet high.

7) We selected answer B because:

1926.452(k) - "Ladder jack scaffolds. "Platforms shall not exceed a height of 20 feet (6.1 m).

All ladders used to support ladder jack scaffolds shall meet the requirements of subpart X of this part -- Stairways and Ladders, except that job-made ladders shall not be used to support ladder jack scaffolds.

The ladder jack shall be so designed and constructed that it will bear on the side rails and ladder rungs or on the ladder rungs alone. If bearing on rungs only, the bearing area shall include a length of at least 10 inches (25.4 cm) on each rung.

8) We selected answer B because:

The OSHA Form 300 must be maintained in the workplace for 5 years. Records of investigation must be maintained for 30 years.

9) We selected answer A because:

The Threshold Limit Value (TLV) as defined by American Conference of Governmental Industrial Hygienists (ACGIH) refer to "airborne concentrations of substance and represent conditions under which it is believed that nearly all workers may be repeatedly exposed day after day without adverse health effects". Certainly information about TLVs should be included in welder training, however this question asked about the fire characteristics of hazardous chemicals. TLVs mainly concern health effects and are not indicators of flammability. Selection "B" autoignition temperature is defined by the National Fire Protection Association (NFPA) as "The lowest temperature at which a flammable gas or vapor-air-mixture will ignite from its own heat source or a contacted heat source without the necessity of spark or flame". Selection "C" the Lower Explosive Limit is defined as "The minimum concentration of combustible gas or vapor in air below which propagation of flame does not occur on contact with a source of ignition". Selection "D" Upper Explosive Limit is defined as "The maximum concentration of vapor or gas in air above which propagation of flame does not occur".

10) We selected answer D because:

Activated charcoal and Silica gel are the most widely used solid sorbent tubes used for air sampling. Activated charcoal is used for organic vapor sampling. It has a large surface area and high adsorptive capacity. It is electrically nonpolar so it prefers organic vapors rather than water vapor. Silica gel is an efficient collector of inorganic substances. It is electrically polar so it prefers water vapor which can seriously interfere with the collection of the contaminant.

11) We selected answer B because:

The NFPA 704 System Hazard Diamond is a symbol system intended for use of fixed installations, such as chemical processing equipment, storage and warehousing rooms and laboratory entrances. It tells a fire fighter what he must do to protect himself from injury while fighting a fire in the area. In this diamond, the three is the fire diamond.

NFPA 704 Symbol

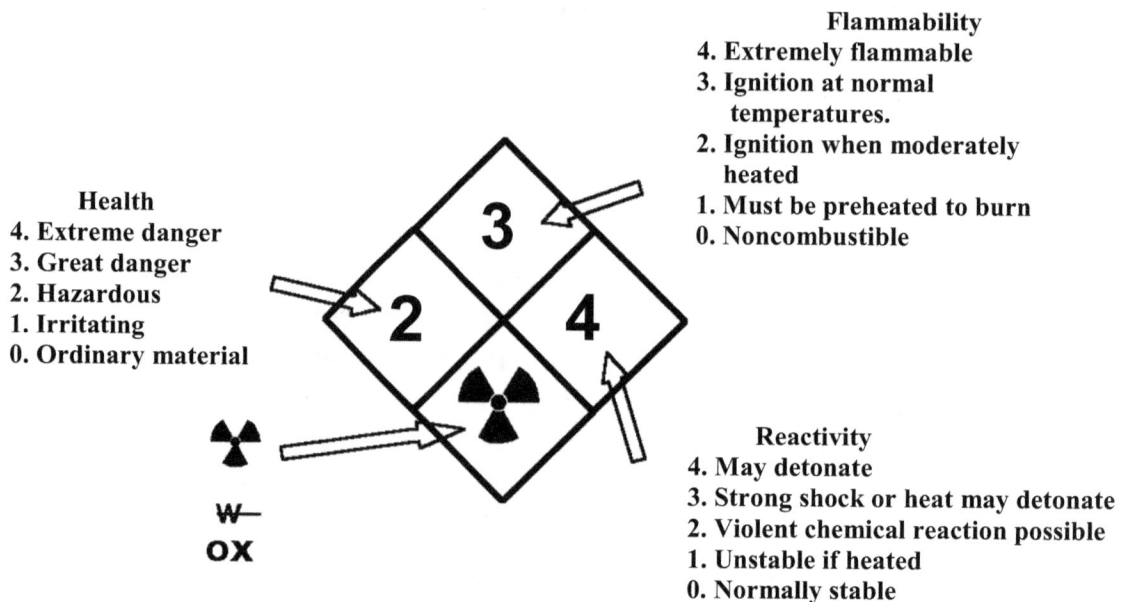

Flammability
4. Extremely flammable
3. Ignition at normal temperatures.
2. Ignition when moderately heated
1. Must be preheated to burn
0. Noncombustible

Health
4. Extreme danger
3. Great danger
2. Hazardous
1. Irritating
0. Ordinary material

W—
OX

Reactivity
4. May detonate
3. Strong shock or heat may detonate
2. Violent chemical reaction possible
1. Unstable if heated
0. Normally stable

12) We selected answer D because:

The Hazard Communication differs from a lot of OSHA standards because it is performance based. This means that you have the flexibility to adapt the rule to the needs of your individual workplace, rather than having to follow specific, rigid requirements. It also means that you have to exercise more judgment to implement an appropriate and effective program. Specification based standards prescribe specific actions to be taken and do not allow any flexibility. One example of a specification standard might be the Mine Safety and Health Administration Standards for miner training. These standards are very specific and outline subjects to be taught, hours required and instructor qualifications.

13) We selected answer D because:

NFPA 101 is the life safety code and is used extensively throughout the United States.

14) We selected answer B because:

Selection "A" is false, training on the OSHA Hazard Communication Standard must be done anytime a new hazard is introduced into the workplace. Selection "B" is the best choice, the MSDSs requirements apply to free samples provided by chemical manufacturers and importers since the hazards remain the same regardless of the cost to the employer. Selection "C" is false, labels must be in English, however, labels and MSDSs may also be in Spanish or another language if desired. In fact, according to OSHA "if employees receive job instructions in a language other than English, then training and information will probably also need to be conducted in a foreign language". Selection "D" is incorrect, MSDSs are considered Employee Exposure and Medical records and as such must be kept 30 years.

15) We selected answer B because:

OSHA requires a competent person to provide training on the nature of fall hazards, the correct procedures for erection, maintenance and disassembly, the proper use, placement and care in handling, etc. Additionally, all erection and disassembly must be done under the supervision of a competent person.

16) We selected answer A because:

The establishment of Training Objectives is the key to good planning. No other single element has the ability to allow the training program to succeed.

17) We selected answer A because:

To be effective, Safety Committees should not be concerned with the day to day activities of the safety program within the company...that is, they should not purchase safety equipment, or investigate minor hazards or accidents. They should be responsible for direction of the overall safety effort and provide guidance for the various program elements.

18) We selected answer D because:

CFR1910.178, Powered Industrial Trucks, requires anyone changing equipment or workplace location to meet the requirements outlined in the Refresher Training requirements (para 1910.178 (l)(4)). Only employees that are trained and authorized should operate industrial powered trucks.

19) We selected answer D because:

According to the NSC, OJT or JIT is widely used because it allows the worker to produce during the training period. The primary instruction is the demonstration or demonstration-performance method of training.

20) We selected answer A because:

According to the NSC, a needs assessment helps to:
- A) Distinguishes between training and non-training needs
- B) Identifies the problem or need before designing a solution
- C) Saves time and money by ensuring that solutions effectively address the problems they are intended to solve
- D) Identifies factors that will impact the training before its development

After the first step in the training process which is the needs assessment, training goals are developed and during that process you will determine what knowledge the trainee needs to know to eliminate the problem. Remember, if you want them to tell time, then teach them how to tell time, not how to build a watch.

21) We selected answer C because:

Job performance is the most effective and final measure of any training program and the training should be designed to correct skill deficiencies. Testing is highly recommended when the effectiveness of the training may be questioned.

22) We selected answer A because:

Some words that should be avoided when writing learning objectives are; know, understand, appreciate, learn, cover, study. It is almost impossible to determine if the student has accomplished those objectives. Some example preferred words are; explain, classify compare, calculate, demonstrate, operate, measure, troubleshoot, analyze, develop, plan.

23) We selected answer A because:

Employee training records maintained under the provisions of 1910.1030, Bloodborne Pathogens, must be retained for three year from the date on which the training occurred.

24) We selected answer A because:

1910.132(f)(1)
The employer shall provide training to each employee who is required by this section to use PPE. Each such employee shall be trained to know at least the following:

- When PPE is necessary;
- What PPE is necessary;
- How to properly don, doff, adjust, and wear PPE;
- The limitations of the PPE; and,
- The proper care, maintenance, useful life and disposal of the PPE.

1910.132(f)(2)
Each affected employee shall demonstrate an understanding of the training specified in paragraph (f)(1) of this section, and the ability to use PPE properly, before being allowed to perform work requiring the use of PPE.

25) We selected answer D because:

According to the National Fire Protection Association Handbook, the NFPA 704, Identification of the Hazards of Materials is a symbol system intended for use on fixed installations or buildings. It tells the fire fighters what they must do to protect themselves. The system is based on the NFPA Standard 704 diamond, which visually presents information on health, flammability, and the self-reactivity hazard of a material. NFPA 704 describes in great detail the hazards and hazard level which the various numbers indicate for the three hazards. Numbers from 0 through 4 are placed in the three upper diamonds to show the degree of hazard present. The 0 indicates the lowest degree of hazard, 4 indicates the highest. The five categories of *health* hazards are presented in the left diamond, which is colored blue. *Fire* hazards are presented in the top diamond, which is colored red. *Reactivity* (stability) hazards are presented in the right diamond, which is colored yellow. Additionally, special information is presented in the bottom diamond, which is colored white, to convey the dangers of high risk materials.

The five degrees of hazard shown above have the following general meaning to fire fighters:

4   Too dangerous to approach with standard fire fighting equipment and procedures. Withdraw and obtain expert advice on how to handle.

3   Fire can be fought using methods intended for extremely hazardous situations, such as unmanned monitors or personal protective equipment, which prevents all bodily contact.

2   Can be fought with standard procedures, but hazards are present which require certain equipment or procedures to handle safety.

1   Nuisance hazards present, which require some care, but standard firefighting procedures can be used.

0   No special hazards, therefore no special measures.

26)   We selected answer B because:

Adults want satisfactory answers to the following questions to accept and apply learning.

1.   Why is it important?
2.   How can I apply it?
3.   How does it work?
4.   What do I need to know?

27)   We selected answer A because:

Group techniques encourage participation from a selected audience. These methods allow trainees to share ideas, evaluate information and become actively involved in the planning and implementation of company policy. Group training is helpful when you need to transfer specific information to a group of people who need to know the same information.

28)   We selected answer A because:

CFR 1910.146 does not require annual training.

"When the employer's permit entry program allows attendant entry for rescue, attendants may enter a permit space to attempt a rescue if they have been trained and equipped for rescue operations as required by paragraph (k)(1) of this section and if they have been relieved as required by paragraph (i)(4) of this section."

29) We selected answer B because:

ISP is the abbreviation for Internet Service Provider and refers to organizations that offer Internet access and data storage services. T-1 is a dedicated phone connection supporting data rates of 1.544Mbits per second. A T-1 line actually consists of 24 individual channels, each of which supports 64Kbits per second.

DSL refers collectively to all types of digital subscriber lines, the two main categories being ADSL and SDSL. Two other types of DSL technologies are *High-data-rate DSL (HDSL)* and *Symmetric DSL (SDSL)*. DSL technologies use sophisticated modulation schemes to pack data onto copper wires. They are sometimes referred to as last-mile technologies because they are used only for connections from a telephone switching station to a home or office, not between switching stations.

POTS is short for plain old telephone service, which refers to the standard telephone service that most homes use. In contrast, telephone services based on high-speed, digital communications lines, such as ISDN and FDDI, are not POTS. The main distinctions between POTS and non-POTS services are speed and bandwidth. POTS is generally restricted to about 52 Kbps (52,000 bits per second).

30) We selected answer B because:

Anthracosis is a pneumoconiosis caused by the exposure to coal dust (black lung). *Silicosis* is a pneumoconiosis caused by inhalation of the dust of stone, sand, or flint containing silica. **Siderosis** is a lung disease caused by inhalation of iron oxide or other metallic particles. *Silicosiderosis* is a pneumoconiosis in which the inhaled dust is that of silica and iron.

31) We selected answer D because:

Interference from other substances in the sample air should always be a primary consideration, because the greatest single source of error in colorimetric sampling is interferences by other contaminants.

32) We selected answer A because:

The practice of interchanging colorimetric tubes is not permitted because it may lead to erroneous results. The primary considerations are the volume of the pump and the rate of the chemical reagents in the indicator tubes.

33) We selected answer C because:

When the vapor pressure of a liquid is greater than the atmospheric pressure the material has reached its boiling point.

34) We selected answer A because:

Supervisors are in the best position to provide realistic and effective training for industrial workers. They have detailed knowledge of work processes and control workflow.

35) We selected answer B because:

Colorimetric tubes provide one of the easiest and least expensive sampling techniques. The tubes use a chemical reaction with the contaminant to create a color change. The amount of color change or the length of the color change is proportional to the vapor or gas concentration. These tubes are not extremely reliable, with an accuracy of about 20 to 50 percent. One severe limitation is cross sensitivity. Often sampling of this type is inaccurate due to interferences caused by other chemicals in the atmosphere. The tubes do have a long shelf life, which can be extended somewhat by storing in a cool dry container.

36) We selected answer B because:

The *Agency of Accident* is the term used in ANSI Z16.2 to identify the object, substance, or premises that contained a hazardous physical condition or circumstance.

37) We selected answer C because:

Colorimetric tubes are relatively cheap, have a fairly long shelf life and are easy to read. Colorimetric or Draeger® Tubes are the most often used measuring device when taking Industrial Hygiene measurements. They do not however provide very precise results, even certified tubes have a plus or minus 25% tolerance.

38) We selected answer D because:

1926.550(g)(5)
A trial lift with the unoccupied personnel platform loaded at least to the anticipated lift weight shall be made from ground level, or any other location where employees will enter the platform to each location at which the personnel platform is to be hoisted and positioned. This trial lift shall be performed immediately prior to placing personnel on the platform. The operator shall determine that all systems, controls and safety devices are activated and functioning properly; that no interferences exist; and that all configurations necessary to reach those work locations will allow the operator to remain under the 50 percent limit of the hoist's rated capacity. Materials and tools to be used during the actual lift can be loaded in the platform, as provided in paragraphs (g)(4)(iii)(D), and (E) of this section for the trial lift. A single trial lift may be performed at one time for all locations that are to be reached from a single set up position. The trial lift shall be repeated prior to hoisting employees whenever the crane or derrick is moved and set up in a new location or returned to a previously used location. Additionally, the trial lift shall be repeated when the lift route is changed unless the operator determines that the route change is not significant (i.e. the route change would not affect the safety of hoisted employees.)

39) We selected answer C because:

1926.251(c)(4)
The following limitations shall apply to the use of wire rope:
An eye splice made in any wire rope shall have not less than three full tucks. However, this requirement shall not operate to preclude the use of another form of splice or connection which can be shown to be as efficient and which is not otherwise prohibited. Except for eye splices in the ends of wires and for endless rope slings, each wire rope used in hoisting or lowering, or in pulling loads, shall consist of one continuous piece without knot or splice. Eyes in wire rope bridles, slings, or bull wires shall not be formed by wire rope clips or knots. Wire rope shall not be used if, in any length of eight diameters, the total number of visible broken wires exceeds 10 percent of the total number of wires, or if the rope shows other signs of excessive wear, corrosion, or defect.

40) We selected answer B because:

1926.350(a)(10)

Oxygen cylinders in storage shall be separated from fuel-gas cylinders or combustible materials (especially oil or grease), a minimum distance of 20 feet (6.1 m) or by a noncombustible barrier at least 5 feet (1.5 m) high having a fire-resistance rating of at least one-half hour.

41)   We selected answer C because:

1926.760(a)(1)

Except as provided by paragraph (a)(3) of this section, each employee engaged in a steel erection activity who is on a walking/working surface with an unprotected side or edge more than 15 feet (4.6 m) above a lower level shall be protected from fall hazards by guardrail systems, safety net systems, personal fall arrest systems, positioning device systems or fall restraint systems.

1926.760(a)(2)

Perimeter safety cables. On multi-story structures, perimeter safety cables shall be installed at the final interior and exterior perimeters of the floors as soon as the metal decking has been installed.

1926.760(a)(3)

Connectors and employees working in controlled decking zones shall be protected from fall hazards as provided in paragraphs (b) and (c) of this section, respectively.

42)   We selected answer A because:

Public Law 91-596, is the Occupational Safety and Health Act. Public Law 91-173, December 30, 1969, was the Federal Coal Mine Health and Safety Act. Public Law 91-577, is the Federal Metal and Non-metallic Mine Safety Act. Public Law 91-173, November 9, 1977, is the Federal Mine Safety and Health Act. The General Duty clause is part of Public Law 91-596 that says "Each employer shall furnish to each of his employees employment and a place of employment which are free from recognized hazards that are causing or likely to cause death or serious physical harm to his employees".

43)   We selected answer A because:

SQL is the abbreviation for Structured Query Language. It is a standardized application language for relational databases that is used to enter data into a database, modify data, delete date and retrieve data.

URL is the abbreviation of Uniform Resource Locator, the global address of documents and other resources on the World Wide Web.

HTML stands for Hyper Text Markup Language and is used for web publishing.

HTTP stands for Hyper Text Transfer Protocol and is a file transfer protocol.

44) We selected answer D because:

The person to correct the hazard should be the individual with the most knowledge of the area, that is the area supervisor.

45) We selected answer D because:

This can be a difficult question, but the BEST answer of those listed it to only make recommendations if you are sure that the result will ensure a safer work area. Making recommendations about areas that you are not skill in has the potential to be incorrect.

46) We selected answer C because:

CM rules are outlined in the Certification Maintenance Guide and it states:

> "A failure to meet your CM requirements results in your OHST or CHST certification being revoked. You may re-acquire the certification by paying the examination fee (reapplication is not required) and passing the current OHST or CHST examination. You must complete this activity within five years of being notified that the certification is no longer valid.

If more than five years passes after losing your OHST or CHST certification because CM requirements were not met, you must seek the certification as a new applicant."

47) We selected answer A because:

The first action should be to contact the supervisor who has control of the workplace and discuss the infraction. Further action may include some of the other solutions presented in the above options.

48) We selected answer C because:
- According to the OSHA policy for determining who gets cited there are three classifications.
- The employer who actually creates the hazard "CREATING EMPLOYER"

- The employer who is responsible, by contract or through actual practice, for safety and health conditions on the worksite; ie, the employer who has the authority for ensuring that the hazardous condition is corrected "CONTROLLING EMPLOYER"
- The employer who has the responsibility for actually correcting the hazard "CORRECTING EMPLOYER"

It must be shown that each employer to be cited has knowledge of the hazardous condition or could have had such knowledge with the exercise of reasonable diligence. In the case cited the sub-contractor would be considered the "creating employer" and the general contractor would be the "controlling employer". In practice it is difficult not to be cited as the controlling employer if you are a general contractor. You must show a defense that satisfies all of the following:

- You did not create the hazard
- You did not have the responsibility or the authority to have the hazard corrected
- You did not have the ability to correct or remove the hazard
- You can demonstrate that the correcting employers, as appropriate, have been specifically notified of the hazards to which his/her employees are exposed
- You have instructed your employees to recognize the hazard and informed them how to avoid the dangers associated with it when the hazard was known or with the exercise of reasonable diligence could have been known

Additionally, in accordance with 1910.132 "Where employees provide their own protective equipment, the employer shall be responsible to assure its adequacy, including proper maintenance, and sanitation of such equipment."

It would appear that in this case both the general contractor and the sub-contractor would receive a citation.

49) We selected answer A because:

When presenting material that is new to a trainee, refrain from asking them to validate the content of the training program. Questions concerning the training environment, the instructor's skill and presentation are valid questions.

50) We selected answer A because:

Progressive companies believe the proper way to deal with minor rule infractions is to issue an oral reprimand for the first offense. Progressive discipline is then administered for additional violations.

51) We selected answer D because:
The controlling employer, in this case the general contractor, will normally be cited if the label or MSDS is not available. However, if the MSDS is not available because the subcontractor failed to provide it, then the subcontractor would instead be cited.

52) We selected answer C because:

Reaction is the least valuable at the end of the training, since the student does not know the actual use of the skills or knowledge gained until they put it into action. That is why most training experts recommend a second critique after six months to obtain a valid reaction from the students.

53) We selected answer B because:
OSHA states "Chemical manufacturers and importers shall evaluate chemicals produced in their workplaces or imported by them to determine if they are hazardous. Employers are not required to evaluate chemicals unless they choose not to rely on the evaluation performed by the chemical manufacturer or importer for the chemical to satisfy this requirement".

54) We selected answer A because:

A Title Act is the method a state would choose to enact specific Title Protection. The purpose of title protection according to an ASSE Position Statement is to "provide legal recognition to the profession of safety as well as provide assurance to the public that individuals representing themselves as being involved in the profession of safety **as safety professionals,** have met the listed minimum qualifications, thereby protecting the public health and safety from harm."
If an individual uses the CHST designation without first being certified by the BCSP, that individual may be barred from pursuing any BCSP certification and/or be sued.

55) We selected answer C because:

Preventative maintenance schedules can be developed from the detailed analysis of a system or process that a Failure Mode and Effects Analysis (FMEA) provides. The analysis provides an indication of which component failure is maintenance dependent as well as how the overall system will benefit from extended life of critical parts.

56) We selected answer D because:

The National Institute for Occupational Safety and Health (NIOSH) is administratively located within the Center for Disease Control (CDC) who functions as a member of the Public Health Service (PHS), which reports to the Department of Health and Human Services (HHS). NIOSH was originally founded within the Department of Health, Education, and Welfare, which is now HHS, under the provisions of the OSHAct. It has prime responsibility for research to eliminate occupational health and safety hazards. NIOSH has the responsibility to identify hazards and recommend changes in the regulations. It performs testing and certification of workers personal protective equipment, mainly respirators. NIOSH has a very active training grant program that supports university training throughout the country and conducts excellent courses at regional centers. NIOSH also does workplace investigations under 42 CFR Part 85, largely to conduct epidemiological methods research and studies. NIOSH does not provide enforcement actions.

57) We selected answer D because:

The operational control delegated the safety engineer to shut down dangerous jobs by the General Manager is functional or line authority. This authority, or lack of it, is hotly debated by safety and health professionals. One position calls the delegation of such power unnecessary. This opinion states that even the threat of a shutdown is most certainly going to be a confrontational issue. An issue that will eventually have to be resolved by higher authority and that often leads to long lasting negative relations between staff and operations.

The other side of this debate feels they need the reserve strength over line managers because of the conflict between organizational demands and safety concerns. They further advance the argument by noting that the act of delegation of authority is in itself a strong commitment by senior management to the safety process.

58) We selected answer B because:

OSHA 1020, Access to employee exposure and medical records, requires that medical records, which includes workplace monitoring records be kept for the duration of employment plus 30 years. There is one exception to the 30-year requirement that affects construction employers. The medical records of employees who have worked for less than one year for the employer need not be retained beyond the term of employment if they are provided to the employee upon termination of employment.

59) We selected answer B because:

The CHST is sponsored by the American Board of Industrial Hygiene and the Board of Certified Safety Professionals.

60) We selected answer B because:

The first term provided in the answers "fire proof" is a contradiction. There is no such thing as fire proof. All known materials will suffer from the effects of a fire if exposed to sufficient intensity and duration.

The second term "fire resistive" is generally considered to include non-combustible. Non-combustible is defined as "not capable of burning or supporting combustion". Fire resistive implies a resistance to an expected fire ie; within design limits. The term is usually used to indicate the ability of a structure or device to withstand the effects of a severe fire for an extended period. Fire resistance is usually indicated in hourly periods determined by standardized fire tests using a time-temperature curve ie; one hour fire wall. Fire resistive is at least one step above non-combustible. Thus, fire resistive materials are always non-combustible but non-combustible materials may not always be fire resistive.

The third choice, "flame proof" is a very ill-defined term the use of which is highly discouraged.

Fire retardant is a useful term indicating a lesser degree of protection than "fire resistive". It is generally used to indicate treated interior and exterior building materials ie; fire retardant plywood. Another term "flame retardant" is also commonly encountered and is used to indicate the treatment of furnishings or decorations. Christmas trees are often treated to be flame retardant.

61) We selected answer D because:

We feel that all of the actions listed will make line supervision take notice. However, a combination of efforts is required to maintain accountability.

62) We selected answer D because:

OSHA construction standards can be found at 29 CFR 1926.

63) We selected answer D because:

The OSHA DART is useful in industrial safety work as an indicator of an accident frequency rate to compare your organization's accident severity and frequency against other similar industry rates.

64) We selected answer D because:

The green triangle with and A is for ordinary combustible fires. B is for flammable liquids. C is electrical equipment. D is for fires involving certain combustible metals. ANSWER D IS THE BEST RESPONSE.

65) We selected answer B because:

The Management by Objective System (MBO) is an excellent method for the employee and supervision to set goals and rate performance.

66) We selected answer C because:

1926.951(c)(1): Portable metal or conductive ladders shall not be used near energized lines or equipment except as may be necessary in specialized work such as in high voltage substations where nonconductive ladders might present a greater hazard than conductive ladders. Conductive or metal ladders shall be prominently marked as conductive and all necessary precautions shall be taken when used in specialized work.

67) We selected answer C because:

The flame symbol on the top indicates a flammable material, the number 1133 is the UN Number and the "3" indicates the hazard class. Examples of UN Numbers are 1033 is for Dimethyl Ether (class 2), 1133 is for Adhesives (class 3) and 1333 is for Cerium (class 4).

68) We selected answer A because:

As a link in the Chain of Custody, that is a person with a duty to preserve and protect evidence or someone with a vested interest in the outcome of the accident investigation, it is essential that from the moment the event occurs you identify, track and log movement of your evidence. An example of Chain of Custody would be taking photos, printing photos, making notes describing the angles that the photo were taken, lighting, date/time, and any other information that could be helpful later in the process.

69) We selected answer A because:

1926.252
Whenever materials are dropped more than 20 feet to any point lying outside the exterior walls of the building, an enclosed chute of wood, or equivalent material, shall be used. For the purpose of this paragraph, an enclosed chute is a slide, closed in on all sides, through which material is moved from a high place to a lower one. When debris is dropped through holes in the floor without the use of chutes, the area onto which the material is dropped shall be completely enclosed with barricades not less than 42 inches high and not less than 6 feet back from the projected edge of the opening above. Signs warning of the hazard of falling materials shall be posted at each level. Removal shall not be permitted in this lower area until debris handling ceases above. All scrap lumber, waste material, and rubbish shall be removed from the immediate work area as the work progresses. Disposal of waste material or debris by burning shall comply with local fire regulations. All solvent waste, oily rags, and flammable liquids shall be kept in fire resistant covered containers until removed from worksite.

70) We selected answer C because:

Local exhaust ventilation almost always costs more than dilution ventilation. Dilution ventilation is defined as the removing or adding of air to keep the concentration of a contaminant below hazardous levels. The process can use natural or forced air movement through open doors, windows, etc. or, exhaust fans can be mounted on roofs, walls, or windows. Local exhaust systems trap the air contaminant near its source which usually makes this method much more effective, but more expensive than dilution. Exhaust Ventilation can be used to remove flammable vapors, mists or powders to a safe location and to confine and control combustible residues.

71)   We selected answer D because:

The range of 70-100 mA is widely accepted as enough current to produce a fatality. Many cases of deaths from low voltages have been reported. Even though CFR 1926 requires GFCIs on all 120 volt, single phase, 15 and 20 amp receptacles on construction sites, the best protection is provided by GFCIs on all 120 and 240 volt receptacles.

72)   We selected answer B because:

Personal protective equipment does decrease injuries however, efficiency is almost always affected. Remember that a single PPE may not always provide adequate protection, for example, you generally have to wear eye protection under a face shield.

1910.132

Application: Protective equipment, including personal protective equipment for eyes, face, head, and extremities, protective clothing, respiratory devices, and protective shields and barriers, shall be provided by the employer, used, and maintained in a sanitary and reliable condition wherever it is necessary by reason of hazards of processes or environment, chemical hazards, radiological hazards, or mechanical irritants encountered in a manner capable of causing injury or impairment in the function of any part of the body through absorption, inhalation or physical contact. Employee-owned equipment: Where employees provide their own protective equipment, the employer shall be responsible to assure its adequacy, including proper maintenance, and sanitation of such equipment.

73)   We selected answer A because:

OSHA 1926.56 requires 5 footcandles for general construction work areas. The table below may offer some assistance, remember the table is for **Minimum Illumination For Safety of Personnel.** For areas or operations not covered in the table, or for illumination levels for efficient visual performance rather than for safety alone refer to ANSI/IES RP7-1983, "Practices for Industrial Lighting", for recommended values. From the table, general construction area lighting should be a minimum of 5 foot candles.

Footcandles	Area of Operation
5	General construction; concrete placement, excavation and waste areas, access ways, active storage areas, loading platforms, refueling, and field maintenance areas.
5	Indoors: warehouses, corridors, hallways, and exit ways.
5	Tunnels, shafts and general underground work areas.
10	General construction plant and shops (batch plants, screening plants, mechanical and electric equipment rooms, carpenter shops, rigging lofts and active storerooms, barracks, toilets.
10	Underground operations involving work at a heading involving drilling, mucking, and scaling.
30	First-aid, stations, infirmaries, and offices.

Remember that receptacles for permanent lighting must be on a circuit separate from that used for temporary lighting.

1926.405(a)(2)(ii)(J)

Extension cord sets used with portable electric tools and appliances shall be of three-wire type and shall be designed for hard or extra-hard usage. Flexible cords used with temporary and portable lights shall be designed for hard or extra-hard usage.
NOTE: The National Electrical Code, ANSI/NFPA 70, in Article 400, Table 400-4, lists various types of flexible cords, some of which are noted as being designed for hard or extra-hard usage. Examples of these types of flexible cords include hard service cord (types S, ST, SO, STO) and junior hard service cord (types SJ, SJO, SJT, SJTO).

74) We selected answer C because:

Total heat load is a combination of the heat produced by the body and the environmental heat the body is exposed to. Working in a *120 degree environment* is certainly a situation that would cause concern but is overshadowed by the heat load of *3500 BTU/hr (1000 kcal/hr)*. Extremely heavy work is about 2000 BTU/hr, a load of 3500 BTU/hr is an obvious, severe hazard. An atmosphere of *13 psia* could be encountered within a wide range of occupations and is not a major concern. *Airflow of one air change every fire minutes* could be acceptable with no other information given. However, it should be noted that the number of air changes is a poor basis for ventilation when environmental control of hazards is required. Airflow measured in "changes per minute" is a concept easily understood, but this rapid understanding coupled with ease of application often allows the real problems (contamination control) to go unabated. When getting a new employ acclimatized to heat for a full workday, it usually takes about 5 days to get the body fully adapted.

75) We selected answer B because:

The ground-fault circuit interrupter (GFCI) is a fast acting device, when even a small amount of current (about 5 milliamp) passes to ground any path other than the proper conductor and in a fraction of a second shuts off the power to the circuit. The GFCI will not sense a line-to-line fault. Construction sites must guard against ground faults either by installing GFCIs or through an assured equipment grounding conductor program. To provide the best protection, use GFCIs on all 120 and 240 volt receptacles.

76) We selected answer C because:

Cylinders are not designed for temperatures in excess of 130 degrees F or 54 degrees C.

77) We selected answer B because:

According to ACGIH, the two methods of controlling airflow distribution are the Balance by Design Method and the Blast Gate Method.

78) We selected answer D because:

In accordance with most manufacturers' recommendations and in keeping with good practice, calibrations should be done at the start of measurements and after completions to insure that all readings are accurate. For all measuring instruments, periodic calibration is the most important factor to ensure reliability.

79) We selected answer B because:

According to the table for Type C soil, 8 x 8 timber is required.

80) We selected answer C because:

According to the table for Type A soil, 8 x 8 timber is required.

81) We selected answer D because:

1926.652(c): Design of support systems, shield systems, and other protective systems. Designs of support systems, shield systems, and other protective systems shall be selected and constructed by the employer or his designee and shall be in accordance with the requirements of paragraph (c)(1); or, in the alternative, paragraph (c)(2); or, in the alternative, paragraph (c)(3); or, i the alternative, paragraph (c)(4) as follows:

1926.652(c)(1): Option (1) - Designs using appendices A, C and D. Designs for timber shoring in trenches shall be determined in accordance with the conditions and requirements set forth in appendices A and C to this subpart. Designs for aluminum hydraulic shoring shall be in accordance with paragraph (c)(2) of this section, but if manufacturer's tabulated data cannot be utilized, designs shall be in accordance with appendix D.

1926.652(c)(4): Option (4) - Design by a registered professional engineer.

1926.652(c)(4)(i): **Support systems, shield systems, and other protective systems not utilizing Option 1, Option 2 or Option 3, above, shall be approved by a registered professional engineer.**

82) We selected answer D because:

The bottom line in any training or education effort is to provide a message that will be understood and acted on by the workers.

83) We selected answer C because:

The following information was extracted from the guidance OSHA provides to OSHA Compliance Safety & Health Officers in the Field Inspection Reference Manual.
Repeated Violations. An employer may be cited for a repeated violation if that employer has been cited previously for a **substantially similar condition** and the citation has become a final order.

- Identical Standard. Generally, similar conditions can be demonstrated by showing that in both situations the identical standard was violated.
EXCEPTION: Previously a citation was issued for a violation of 29

CFR §1910.132(a) for not requiring the use of safety- toe footwear for employees. A recent inspection of the same establishment revealed a violation of 29 CFR §1910.132(a) for not requiring the use of head protection (hard hats). Although the same standard was involved, the hazardous conditions found were not substantially similar and therefore a repeated violation would not be appropriate.

- Different Standards. In some circumstances, similar conditions can be demonstrated when different standards are violated. Although there may be different standards involved, the hazardous conditions found could be substantially similar and therefore a repeated violation would be appropriate.

- Time Limitations. Although there are no statutory limitations upon the length of time that a citation may serve as a basis for a repeated violation, the following policy shall be used in order to ensure uniformity.

  (a) A citation will be issued as a repeated violation if:

  1 The citation is issued within 5 years of the final order of the previous citation, or,

  2 The citation is issued within 5 years of the final abatement date of that citation, whichever is later.

  (b) When a violation is found during an inspection, and a repeated citation has been issued for a substantially similar condition, which meets the above time limitations, the violation may be classified as a second instance repeated violation with a corresponding increase in penalty.

  (c) For any further repetition, the Area Director shall be consulted for guidance.

Additionally, OSHA has the capability to obtain a national inspection history on employers who operate in several locations. That means they can find all of the citations your company has ever been issued. If you have been issued a citation anywhere within the 5 year time limit, you can be cited for a repeat. If OSHA does not go to the trouble to run a national inspection check you will only be cited for a repeat if the second citation occurs within the same OSHA Area Office jurisdiction.

84) We selected answer C because:

When an establishment has changed ownership, the employer is responsible for maintaining records and filing reports only for that period of the year during which he owned the company. However, in the case of a change in ownership, the employer must preserve the records of the prior ownership. The records belong to the establishment to which they relate.

85) We selected answer A because:

First aid treatment is defined by OSHA as "any one-time treatment, and any follow-up visit for the purpose of observation, of minor scratches, cuts, burns, splinters, and so forth, which do not ordinarily require medical care. Such one-time treatment, and follow-up visit for the purpose of observation, is considered first aid even though provided by a physician or registered professional personnel."

86) The best selection is answer A because:

According to the OSHA Hazard Communication Standard (29 CFR 1926.59) employers shall provide employees with information and training on hazardous chemicals in their work area:

- at time of initial assignment
- if transferred to a new assignment with new chemical hazards
- when a new chemical hazard is introduced into the work place

87) The best selection is answer C because

According to the National Safety Council publication *Basics of Safety and Health,* common methods of hazard control, in order of precedence, are: designing out the hazard, eliminating the hazard by substitution or automation, reducing exposure, and using personal protective equipment.

88) The best selection is answer D because:

Installation of anti-two-blocking device does not affect the load capacity of a mobile crane.

89) The best selection is answer C because:

Although all of the answer choices are plausible causes, they may be indirect. An equipment malfunction is the best representation of a direct cause.

90) We selected Answer D because:

The following information was extracted from the Hazard Communication Standard "QUIP" published by OSHA. In response to a request for clarification OSHA stated "If it is determined that an employee has not received training or is not adequately trained, the current employer will be held responsible regardless of who provided the training to the employee. An employer, therefore, has a responsibility to evaluate an employee's level of knowledge with regard to the training and information requirements of the standard, and the employer's own hazard communication program, including previous training the employee may have received."

91) We selected answer C because:

According to The NFPA Fire Protection Handbook, for combustion to occur, four components are necessary: Oxygen (oxidizing agent); Fuel(substrate); Heat(ignition); and a self-sustained chemical reaction (also referred to as the chain reaction). These components can be graphically described as the "fire tetrahedron". Each component of the tetrahedron must be in place for combustion to occur. Remove any one of the four components and combustion will not occur. If ignition has already occurred, the fire is extinguished when one of the components is removed from the reaction.

92) We selected answer A because:

According to the Fundamental of Industrial Hygiene, an Industrial Toxicologist is one who studies the harmful, or toxic, properties of substances and determine dose thresholds. An Industrial Hygienist is one devoted to the art and science of anticipation, recognition, evaluation and control of those environmental factors in the workplace that may cause sickness, impaired health and well being. A Health Physicist studies the field of science concerned with radiation physics and radiation biology with the goal of providing technical information and proper techniques regarding the safe use of ionizing radiation. Pathologists are physicians who diagnose and characterize disease in living patients by examining biopsies or bodily fluid. Pathologists may also conduct autopsies to investigate causes of death.

93) We selected answer C because:

In Roger Brauer's *Safety and Health for Engineers*, before forwarding a recommendation for corrective action to train (or retrain) employees, a safety professional should check to see if one or more effective engineering controls would cost effectively reduce the risk to an acceptable level.

94) We selected answer D because:

As referenced in by the Center for Chemical Process Safety *Guidelines for Hazard Evaluation Procedures,* 2nd Edition, subject matter experts familiar with the process being studied are essential. A process hazard analysis leader familiar with the analytical method is important, but it is not essential for the study leader to be personally familiar with the actual process being studied.

95) We selected answer C because:

In the book *Safety Culture and Effective Safety Management,* author Swartz explains that before collecting data and developing a system to collect and manipulate the data, it is essential to define how the data will be used.

96) We selected answer C because:

A pocket dosimeter measures a person's accumulated radiation dose. A pocket dosimeter is frequently used in conjunction with a film badge (themoluminescent dosimetry badge).

97) We selected answer C because:

The *Accident Prevention Manual for Business and Industry: Engineering and Technology,* 12th Edition, National Safety Council explains that Electric arc welding produces ozone (O_3), a hazardous gas

98) We selected answer A because:

In *Accident Prevention Manual for Business and Industry: Administration and Programs,* A key part of risk management is investigating incidents and taking corrective actions based upon the facts associated with the incidents. An essential aspect of the investigation process is understanding the causal factors and the subsequent root causes that had to the incidents so appropriate corrective actions can be identified and implemented.

99) We selected answer C because:

According to *Developing Safety Training Programs,* A learning objective must identify what the student will be able to do at the end of the training program. It is not part of the outline of the training program.

100) We selected Answer D because

According to Peterson's Techniques of Safety Management, only answers A, B, and C are representative of basic principles of loss control.

CPSIA information can be obtained
at www.ICGtesting.com
Printed in the USA
FSHW021758030320
67775FS